End Stage Therapy and Heart Transplantation

Edited by Norihide Fukushima

Published in London, United Kingdom

End Stage Therapy and Heart Transplantation
http://dx.doi.org/10.5772/intechopen.111188
Edited by Norihide Fukushima

Contributors
Füsun Afşar, Abdulwahid Almulla, Ali Kindawi, Amr Salah Omar, Brisha Best, Chawannuch Ruaengsri, Chidiebere Peter Echieh, Daniel M. Bethencourt, Daniel Zimpfer, Dina Fa Alwaheidi, Hideki Ito, Kamen Dimitrov, Kulpreet Barn, Masato Mutsuga, Michael Sobieraj, Norihide Fukushima, Robert Hooker, Sabaa Ahmed, Sankar Balasubramanian, Sho Akita, Stephen Crawford, Tamer Abdalghafoor, Tiffany Koyano, Toshiaki Akita, Toshiya Sasaki, Yasuhiro Shudo

First published in London, United Kingdom, 2024 by IntechOpen
IntechOpen is the global imprint of INTECHOPEN LIMITED, registered in England and Wales, registration number: 11086078, 167-169 Great Portland Street, London, W1W 5PF, United Kingdom

British Library Cataloguing-in-Publication Data
A catalogue record for this book is available from the British Library

Additional hard and PDF copies can be obtained from orders@intechopen.com

End Stage Therapy and Heart Transplantation
Edited by Norihide Fukushima
p. cm.

This title is part of the Cardiology and Cardiovascular Medicine Book Series, Volume 2
Topic: Cardiovascular Surgery
Series Editor: Kaan Kırali
Topic Editor: Takashi Murashita

Print ISBN 978-0-85014-171-9
Online ISBN 978-0-85014-172-6
eBook (PDF) ISBN 978-0-85014-173-3
ISSN 3033-361X

For EU product safety concerns:
IN TECH d.o.o., Prolaz Marije Krucifikse Kozulić 3, 51000 Rijeka, Croatia,
info@intechopen.com or visit our website at intechopen.com.

IntechOpen Book Series
Cardiology and Cardiovascular Medicine
Volume 2

Aims and Scope of the Series

Today, since molecular science on structural causes of oncological pathologies and their molecular treatments are developing at an unbelievable rate, the primary medical cause of death in the twenty-first century will be cardiovascular disease. Neither pandemics that threaten all humanity nor deterioration in the ecosystem will be able to change this fact. Especially, this century seems poised to witness an incredible struggle against atherosclerotic disease, which develops in the arterial walls and results in narrowing and occlusion of the arterial lumen. In addition to this disease, there has been an increasing prevalence of heart rhythm problems, deterioration of heart valves due to aging, and heart failure. Serious vascular pathologies such as stenosis and occlusion, dissection and rupture, and aneurysmal enlargement are also major concerns. Medical and invasive treatment methods may work to save human lives, but they will never provide a real solution. All kinds of medical, technological, and genetic engineering developments obtained in these processes have not yet been sufficient to alleviate or eliminate cardiovascular disease. This book series, Cardiology and Cardiovascular Medicine, includes three topics. The first, Cardiovascular Diseases and Health, reviews important cardiovascular diseases and the developments in their prognosis. The second topic, Cardiovascular Electrophysiology, illuminates the abnormal functioning of the cardiac conduction system, which is caused by all heart pathologies and negatively affects prognosis. The third topic in this series, Cardiovascular Surgery, details treatment for cardiovascular pathologies and how to regulate normal physiological functions with percutaneous or extracorporeal interventions.

Meet the Series Editor

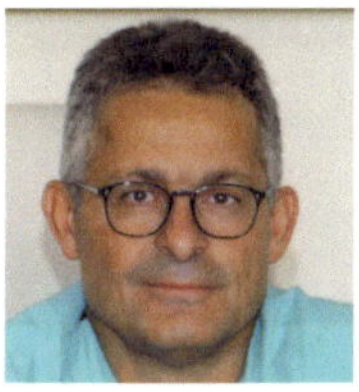

After completing his studies at the Medicine Faculty of Istanbul University in 1990, Prof. Kaan Kırali fulfilled his mandatory medical service and commenced his residency training at Koşuyolu Heart and Research Hospital in 1992. Following five years of assistant education, he pursued further training in England and the USA in 1998. Specializing in laparoscopic and minimally invasive cardiac surgery, he earned the titles of consultant cardiovascular surgeon in 1998, Assistant Professor in 1999, Associate Professor in 2002, and Chief in 2005 at the same hospital. Prof. Kırali also developed an interest in preventive medicine, obtaining an MSc in Public Health from Istanbul University in 2000. Over the past two decades, he has concentrated his scientific pursuits on cardiovascular repairs requiring specialized experience. With his expertise in coronary artery surgery, minimally invasive cardiac surgery, valve repair, and aortic root surgery, he has established new methods for awake coronary bypass revascularization, a new surgical approach for AVR during first and re-operations, aortic valve-sparing procedure, and radiofrequency ablation. Notably, he pioneered awake complete coronary artery bypass grafting (CABG) with bilateral internal mammary arteries (BIMA) and played a crucial role in advancing aortic root surgery with a new aortotomy incision, simplifying aortic valve interventions. Since the year 2000, Prof. Kırali has expanded his interests to heart transplantation, and in recent years, to left ventricular assist devices. He has served as the head of the transplantation department since 2015 and currently continues his work as the director of Koşuyolu High Specialization Education and Research Hospital in Istanbul, Turkey. In his prolific career, he has authored numerous papers in SCI journals, contributed to various book chapters, and served as an editor and reviewer for multiple academic journals. Additionally, he has edited several international books in the field of cardiovascular medicine.

Meet the Volume Editor

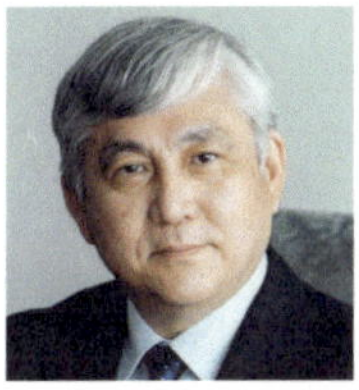

Dr. Norihide Fukushima is a Professor and President of Senri Kinran University Graduate School of Nursing, Japan, a Visiting Director at the National Cerebral and Cardiovascular Center, and a Recruit Professor at the Department of Surgery, Osaka University Graduate School of Medicine, Japan. After graduating from Osaka University Medical School, Dr. Fukushima finished clinical training in the 1st Department of Surgery, Osaka University Hospital, and obtained his Ph.D. in Prolonged Cardiac Immerse Storage in 1992. Dr. Fukushima worked at Loma Linda University, USA as a research and clinical fellow from 1991 to 1994. His team performed the first heart transplantation in Japan in 1999. He and his colleagues revised the Transplant Act in 2010 to increase deceased organ donation and heart transplantation in Japan. He has been working to develop therapeutic strategies for advanced heart failure, such as mechanical circulatory support and medical care.

Contents

Preface

Since the first heart transplantation was performed by Dr. Christiaan Barnard in South Africa in 1967 [1], there has been steady progress in terms of recipient selection, donor selection and management, surgical technique, preoperative management, and immunosuppression regimen as well as mechanical circulatory support during the wait for heart transplantation. The rapid progress in these areas is associated with steady improvement in outcomes before and after heart transplantation.

Medical therapy, including self-care management, has greatly improved outcomes in end-stage heart failure patients who will not receive heart transplants. A cardiac reshaping net for dilated cardiomyopathy is currently being investigated as an alternative method for heart transplantation.

The development of mechanical circulatory support has also changed therapeutic strategies for stage D heart failure patients. After the first total artificial heart as a bridge to transplant (BTT) was done at the Texas Heart Institute in 1972 [2], the extracorporeal left ventricular assist device (LVAD) was introduced to BTT in 1978 and the Novacor LVAD (Baxter Health Corp., Oakland, CA) was first implanted for BTT at Stanford University [3]. The Randomized Evaluation of Mechanical Assistance for the Treatment of Congestive Heart Failure (REMATCH) study [4] revealed that implantable pulsatile LVAD had clinically meaningful survival benefits and improved quality of life in Stage D heart failure patients in 1999; thus, destination therapy took off worldwide.

This book includes eight chapters that provide recent evolutive information on end-stage therapy and heart transplantation.

The "Advanced Heart Failure" section includes Chapter 1, "Self-Care of Patients with Advanced Stage Heart Failure", and Chapter 2, "Cardiac Reshaping Net for Dilated Cardiomyopathy".

The "Mechanical Circulatory Support" section includes Chapter 3, "Extracorporeal Membrane Oxygenation (ECMO) Use in Heart Transplantation", Chapter 4, "Exploring Standard and Alternative Sites for Left Ventricular Assist Device Inflow Cannula and Outflow Graft Placement", and Chapter 5, "LVAD Continuing Care: A Comprehensive Guide to Long-Term Support and Management".

The final section on "Heart Transplantation" includes Chapter 6, "Establishing a Heart Transplantation Program in a Middle East Country: Requirements, Logistics, and Implementation Strategies", Chapter 7, "Heart Preservation Techniques for Transplantation", and Chapter 8, "Heart Transplantation and Mechanical Circulatory Support in Japan – Past, Current and Future Aspects".

I would also like to thank all the contributors for their help in making this special book useful and interesting.

Norihide Fukushima
Professor,
Senri Kinran University Graduate School of Nursing,
Suita, Japan

Visiting Director,
National Cerebral and Cardiovascular Center,
Suita, Japan

References

[1] Cooper DK. Christiaan Barnard and his contributions to heart transplantation. The Journal of Heart and Lung Transplantation. 2001;**20**(6):599-610

[2] Cooley DA. Heart substitution: Transplantation and total artificial heart. The Texas Heart Institute experience. Artificial Organs. 1985;**9**(1):12-16

[3] Starnes VA, Oyer PE, Portner PM, et al. Isolated left ventricular assist as bridge to cardiac transplantation. The Journal of Thoracic and Cardiovascular Surgery. 1988;**96**(1):62-71

[4] Rose EA, Moskowitz AJ, Packer M, et al. The REMATCH trial: Rationale, design, and end points. Randomized Evaluation of Mechanical Assistance for the Treatment of Congestive Heart Failure. The Annals of Thoracic Surgery. 1999;**67**(3):723-730

Section 1

Advanced Heart Failure

Chapter 1

Self-Care of Patients with Advanced Stage Heart Failure

Füsun Afşar

Abstract

Despite continuing scientific and technological developments in the field of healthcare, heart failure has increasing prevalence and incidence throughout the world and remains one of the most important causes of morbidity and mortality. According to the 2015 data of the American Heart Association, there were approximately 6.2 million heart failure patients aged >20 years in the USA, and when 870,00 new diagnoses per year are added, it is estimated that the rate of diagnosed cases will increase by 46% by the year 2030. As heart failure is a chronic and progressive disease, it requires many years of follow-up, treatment, and care. The primary aims of heart failure treatment are to reduce mortality and hospital admissions, increase functional capacity, correct symptoms and findings, and improve quality of life. In addition to the medical treatment of patients with heart failure, to provide compliance with the recommendations related to the management of signs and symptoms which cause mild-severe impairments in daily life because of fatigue, shortness of breath, and other cardiac findings, it is necessary to record and strengthen self-care practices. Self-care is essential for patients with heart failure [HF], and improving self-care is a major focus of multidisciplinary HF management programmes worldwide. This chapter will consider self-care in four phases, determining the self-care evaluation, self-care maintenance, self-care monitoring, and self-care management.

Keywords: heart failure, self-care, evaluation, maintenance, monitoring, management

1. Introduction

Throughout the world, non-infectious diseases are the cause of most deaths and disability, diminish quality of life, and create high healthcare costs. According to 2022 data of the World Health Organisation [WHO], cardiovascular diseases are the leading cause of death [17.9 million deaths] among non-infectious diseases. Heart failure is a syndrome that is dealt within the scope of cardiovascular diseases with a high comorbidity profile, which affects 26 million people worldwide.

Despite continuously developing science and technology in the healthcare sector, heart failure has a high prevalence in older adults and has a negative effect on survival [1]. According to the 2015 data of the American Heart Association, there were approximately 6.2 million patients aged over 20 years with heart failure disease; 870,000 new diagnoses were added every year, and it was predicted that the rate of diagnosis would increase by 46% by 2030 [2]. The prevalence of heart failure in developed countries has been reported to be approximately 1–2% of the adult population and ≥ 10% in those aged >70 years.

The 5- and 10-year survival rates of heart failure patients are 44.5 and 24.5%, respectively. These patients also have frequent hospital admissions. It has been reported that the re-admission rate within 30 days of hospital discharge is 20–30%, and the rehospitalisation rates within the first 6 and 12 months are 28 and 31%, respectively [3]. Heart failure survival has improved over time, but the absolute 5-year mortality rate for heart rate from the time of diagnosis remains at 50%. It has been stated that the financial burden of the care of heart failure patients exceeds 30 million USD per year [4]. The estimation of the prevalence of advanced stage heart failure continues to be an epidemiological difficulty as a result of the relatively low incidence of this condition and the dependence of detection on a developing range of treatments [5].

2. Advanced heart failure

2.1 The identification and classification of advanced stage heart failure

Advanced stage heart disease is a process that significantly reduces quality of life and survival, in which more serious signs and heart failure symptoms continue during mild effort and/or at rest despite optimal evidence-based medical treatment, device treatment, or surgical intervention and which requires several important decisions to be taken in management of the disease such as frequent re-admission to hospital, the need for inotropic treatment, and the placement of mechanical support devices or heart transplantation [6].

Since heart failure is a progressive syndrome, the necessity of evaluating the functional capacity and symptoms of the patients is also at the forefront. When the classification systems used to define the severity of HF are examined, it is seen that the American College of Cardiology [ACC] also includes the risk factors in the classification, and the New York Heart Association [NYHA] is a classification system based on functional status [7].

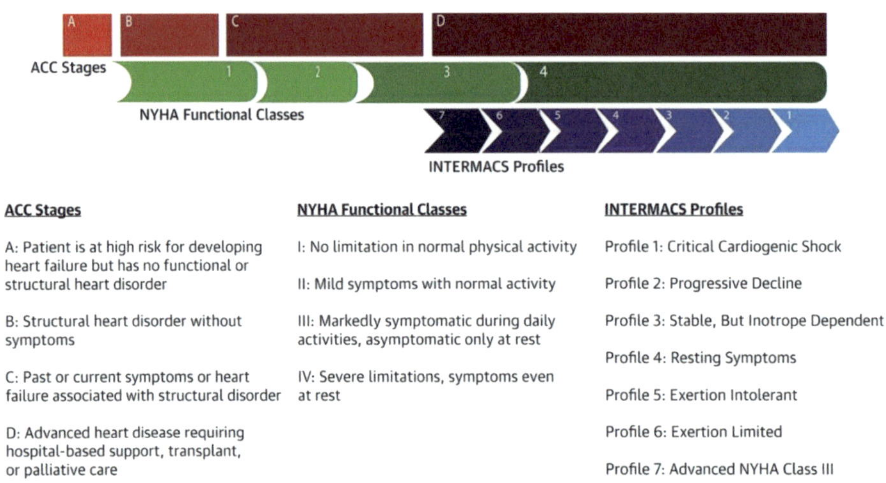

Figure 1.
Advanced stage heart disease classification [7].

In various studies, advanced stage heart disease has been identified most often with the two measurements of left ventricle ejection fraction [generally <35%] and low functional capacity [NYHA III-IV]. Currently, the most appropriate classification system to answer the question of "at what stage of advanced heart failure does the patient require a mechanical support device or heart transplantation treatment?" is the INTERMACS classification (**Figure 1**) [8].

2.2 Advanced heart failure symptoms

Advanced stage heart failure has been defined as a syndrome requiring the presence of at least a few of the cardinal symptoms such as shortness of breath, fluid retention/oedema, fatigue, activity intolerance, and exercise limitations [9]. The aetiology of symptoms in heart failure is complex and difficult to understand. These symptoms are partly due to an increase in left ventricle filling pressure, partly due to a decrease in cardiac flow rate, and partly due to widespread myopathy (**Table 1**) [8].

Shortness of breath seen associated with pulmonary congestion that develops due to heart failure is the most common symptom of heart failure. Exercise dyspnoea, orthopnoea, and paroxysmal nocturnal dyspnoea are among the symptoms seen in advanced heart failure in particular, and these affect physiological processes in all tissues [10]. Therefore, the grading of dyspnoea and evaluation of accompanying symptoms are important in symptom management. In addition to medical treatment in dyspnoea management, respiratory exercises are used in mild- and moderate-level dyspnoea, and positive pressure support devices are used in the management of advanced grade dyspnoea [11].

Symptoms of heart failure
Typical
Breathlessness
Orthopnoea
Paroxysmal nocturnal dyspnoea
Reduced exercise tolerance
Ankle swelling
Inability to exercise
Swelling of parts of the body other than ankles
Bendopnoea
Less typical
Nocturnal cough
Wheezing
Bloated feeling
Postprandial satiety
Loss of appetite
Decline in cognitive function, confusion [especially in the elderly]
Depression
Dizziness. Syncope

Table 1.
Advanced stage heart failure symptoms.

Increased activation of inflammatory cytokines creates a catabolic condition resulting in insulin resistance, anorexia, and weight loss. By causing atrophy and weakness in both skeletal and respiratory muscles, this condition further increases physical limitation. In addition, fatigue is one of the frequently seen symptoms in advanced heart failure for reasons such as electrolyte imbalance, overuse of diuretics, thyroid dysfunction, anaemia, and impairment in peripheral oxygenation as a result of a decrease in cardiac circulation and an increase in peripheral vascular resistance. The determination of effort and functional capacity and the monitoring of heart rate and heart rhythm are important in advanced stage heart failure patients [12]. Peripheral oedema seen as systemic venous congestion, abdominal ascites, and fullness in the jugular veins is among the cardinal symptoms in advanced stage heart disease patients. Follow-up of patient weight and the grading of oedema are important in respect of arranging treatment. It is recommended in the ESC 2016 guidelines that patients inform the healthcare team of an unexpected weight increase of more than 2 kg in 3 days [13].

Symptoms such as shortness of breath, lethargy, and fatigue experienced by patients with heart failure because of the nature of the disease itself, and sleep problems and a decrease in sleep quality, which is a basic component of daily living activities, occur because of the drugs used in treatment and limited functional capacity. Sleep disorders such as difficulty in falling asleep and maintaining sleep, insomnia, sleep apnoea syndrome, and excessive daytime sleepiness are frequently seen in individuals with heart failure [14]. Sleep apnoea is the most common cause of sleep disorders seen in heart failure patients. Two types of sleep apnoea are seen: obstructive, as a result of upper respiratory tract collapse, and central, as a decrease in central respiratory stimulus [15].

Comorbid problems and symptoms, especially in elderly patients with advanced heart failure, have a negative effect on the quality of life of patients and lead to frequent hospital admissions. The problems experienced cause depression, anxiety, and feelings of hopelessness in both the patient and their primary caregiver. In the management of psychological symptoms, it is recommended in the ESC 2016 guidelines that the management of self-care is included in the self-care practices of the patient and carers, and when necessary, referral to specialists should be made for mental health support.

Heart failure patients tend to have impaired cognitive functions, and this reduces their capacity to perceive when the disease is worsening and makes compliance with complex heart failure treatments more difficult.

2.3 Advanced stage heart failure treatment

Heart failure treatments include following a healthy lifestyle, drug treatments, operations, and medical support devices.

In the guidelines created by heart failure specialists, pharmacological treatments include diuretics, ACE [angiotensin-converting enzyme inhibitors]/ARB[angiotensin receptor blockers]/ARNI[angiotensin receptor-neprilysin inhibitor], Betablockers, Mineralocorticoid Receptor Antagonists [MRAs], Sodium-Glucose Co-transporter-2 inhibitors, Hydralazine and isosorbide dinitrate, and Digoxin. Regular follow-up of multiple drug use is required for the adjustment of drug doses according to present and developing symptoms [13].

In patients with advanced heart failure, compliance with the drug regimen and the development of lifestyle behaviours such as a low-sodium diet, regular exercise, and monitoring of weight together with the follow-up of drug-related symptoms that could develop are a part of the treatment [16].

When these methods are not sufficient in the treatment of advanced stage heart failure, the patients are evaluated for cardiac support devices [ventricle assistive devices] and heart transplantation.

Based on the European Cardiology Association guidelines for the diagnosis and treatment of acute and chronic heart failure, a commitment to self-care is an important component in improving patient results.

3. Self-care

"Self-care" is defined by the World Health Organisation [WHO] as the ability of individuals, their families, and society to develop health, prevent disease, protect health, and be able to cope with disease and disability with or without the support of healthcare services [17].

The concept of self-care includes the promotion and development of health, prevention and control of disease, self-treatment with drugs, and the provision of care by those on whom the patient is dependent and the participation of healthcare professionals when necessary.

The most important step in the development of self-care is the assessment of the patient. A holistic assessment of the self-care status of a patient and determination of priority areas for behavioural change can provide encouragement and useful basic data for personal change.

Self-care allows individuals to deal with their requirements holistically.

3.1 World Health Organisation self-care behaviours

The World Health Organisation [WHO] has defined self-care behaviours for the maintenance and development of health (**Figure 2**) [17].

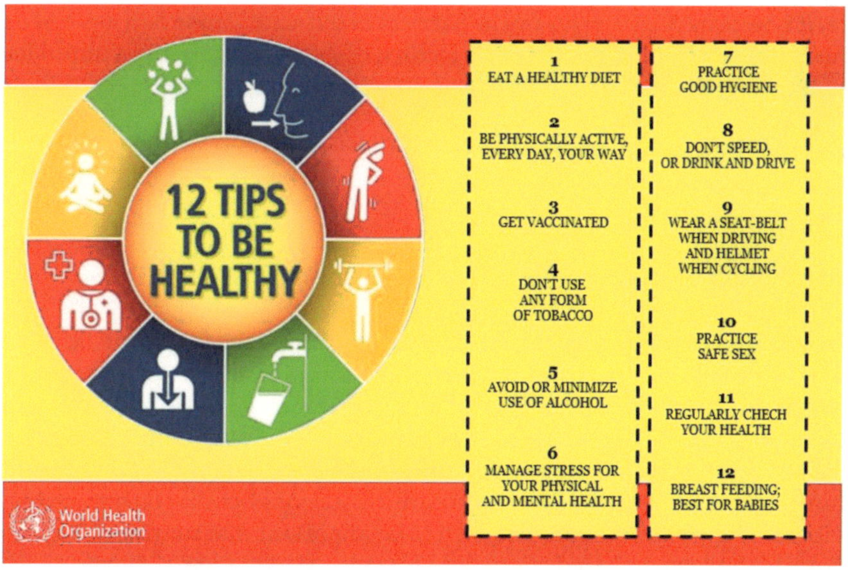
12 TIPS TO BE HEALTHY
1 EAT A HEALTHY DIET
2 BE PHYSICALLY ACTIVE, EVERY DAY, YOUR WAY
3 GET VACCINATED
4 DON'T USE ANY FORM OF TOBACCO
5 AVOID OR MINIMIZE USE OF ALCOHOL
6 MANAGE STRESS FOR YOUR PHYSICAL AND MENTAL HEALTH
7 PRACTICE GOOD HYGIENE
8 DON'T SPEED, OR DRINK AND DRIVE
9 WEAR A SEAT-BELT WHEN DRIVING AND HELMET WHEN CYCLING
10 PRACTICE SAFE SEX
11 REGULARLY CHECH YOUR HEALTH
12 BREAST FEEDING; BEST FOR BABIES
World Health Organization

Figure 2.
Health-promotion tips for self-care practices.

3.2 Maintaining self-care

This has been defined as the process of practices promoting the maintenance of the physical and psychological balance and protecting health through disease management. The requirements of self-care can be listed as health literacy, self-awareness, a moderate level of physical activity, a healthy diet, avoiding or minimising risk, disease knowledge, drug compliance, and rational use of devices related to the treatment.

3.3 Monitoring self-care

Self-care is performed by making judgments from the recording of systematic observations of the individuals, their daily behaviours, their surroundings, and their personal relationships and then comparing their own behaviours with those of others or ideal behaviours.

3.4 Management of self-care

Following the observations and judgement, individuals can identify their own behavioural or environmental problems, and then, by changing behaviours, adjusting the environment, and increasing self-reactions, an appropriate reaction can be given to reach personal targets. Self-care management includes all the activities made by patients to identify and interpret their own symptoms and to manage their own health.

4. Self-care in advanced stage heart failure

Heart failure self-care is defined as the process of health care and disease management, which maintains stability in decisions and behaviours, defined by changes in the patient status and provided by correct applications.

To be able to maintain healthy self-care in patients with advanced stage heart failure, it is necessary to first know the barriers to self-care. These barriers can be examined under 3 headings as personal factors, disease burden, and an unproductive support system [18].

4.1 Factors affecting self-Care in Heart Failure

4.1.1 Personal factors

4.1.1.1 Lack of self-care information

The first step in preventing barriers to poor health outcomes that can be experienced by heart failure patients is for patients and carers to have knowledge at a level that will enable them to adopt and maintain a complex series of behavioural changes.

The reasons for a lack of knowledge of advanced stage heart failure patients and their carers include low education levels, limited health literacy, and education programmes that are presented by healthcare institutions but that do not establish behavioural changes. It has been reported to be important that sources of information are accessible and are prepared taking into consideration the age, sight and hearing impairments, forgetfulness, and low health literacy levels of patients with heart failure, and that regular medical visits are made by healthcare professionals [19].

4.1.1.2 Negative emotions related to heart failure

In addition to sustaining optimistic feelings by hoping that life will be prolonged with evidence-based drug treatments, devices, or surgical options, the culture and beliefs of patients, complex treatments, the presence of symptoms, disability, and negative developments in the disease process can cause negative feelings such as a sense of uncertainty, anxiety, and fear in many patients with advanced heart failure. Emotions such as hopelessness, depression, and anger experienced by heart failure patients can constitute a significant barrier to the self-care process by creating feelings of a lack of interest in life and preferring death to life [18].

4.1.1.3 Difficulties in changing habits

With the determination of personal behaviours that create an increase in disease risk, lifestyle behaviours have entered the agenda of many international institutions such as the European Cardiology Association, the American Diabetes Association, and the WHO. In 2019, the WHO published a self-care behaviours guide for health and well-being. Improvements in self-care have been brought about together with a change in habits.

A diagnosis of heart failure brings lifestyle changes such as disease-specific diet, perception and management of symptoms, drugs, regular medical check-ups, and exercise. Studies of patients with heart failure have reported that patients maintain self-care activities when symptoms become more severe or when they are hospitalised, but then return to previous habits when symptoms are alleviated or after discharge from hospital [20].

4.1.2 Disease burden

The life of a patient with advanced stage heart failure in particular is affected physically, psychologically, economically, socially, and financially, and all these reasons constitute a great burden for patients and carers. The factors affecting the disease burden can be examined in 3 subcategories of physical decline, comorbidities, and financial pressure [2].

4.1.2.1 Progressive physical decline

The symptoms of advanced stage heart failure generally include shortness of breath during exercise or at rest, orthopnoea, lack of energy, fatigue, anorexia, weight loss, depression, sleep disorders, pain, and cognitive disorders [8]. Decreasing physical ability causes difficulties in daily living activities, or lethargy, fatigue and shortness of breath during activities, thereby affecting patients psychologically.

4.1.2.2 Comorbidities

Comorbidities such as hypertension, diabetes mellitus, respiratory problems, osteoarthritis, and gastrointestinal disorders affect the self-care process. As the management of advanced heart failure and comorbidities requires the referral of patients to more than one different medical branch, different laboratory tests, and many drugs to be taken, it is a difficult and tiring process. As each disease has its own dynamics, this makes it difficult for patients to manage the symptoms and comply with treatment [19].

4.1.2.3 Financial pressure

The process of managing advanced heart failure, especially when there are additional comorbidities, creates a financial burden for patients and their primary carers. In addition to the costs of accessing healthcare services, periodic doctor visits, laboratory tests, drugs, specific diets, and frequent hospitalisations, there may also be loss of employment. The fall in income and increased outgoings during the course of the disease can limit the capabilities of patients for self-care [3].

4.1.3 Inadequate support systems

The third main category of barriers to self-care of patients with advanced heart failure is inadequate support systems. There are three subcategories of insufficient social support, lack of attention to self-care by healthcare providers, and limited access to healthcare providers.

4.1.3.1 Insufficient social support

Both the presence of symptoms and the treatment of advanced stage heart failure require a long and tiring process. There is a need in this process for family, state, healthcare, and social support in physical, psychosocial, and financial aspects [3].

4.1.3.2 Lack of attention to self-care by healthcare providers

The starting point of self-care is healthcare centres and healthcare professionals in the centre. For the patient to be able to perform effective self-care, healthcare professionals should enable the patient to systematically apply awareness and knowledge. Specialisation in the field of advanced stage heart failure is an important criterion for healthcare professionals undertaking the provision of effective self-care [21].

The main reasons for the lack of attention to self-care by healthcare professionals in the hospital environment are a heavy workload, limited professional autonomy, a medical treatment-focused approach, a limited time for patient education, and a lack of comprehensive hospital discharge programmes. The responsibilities of healthcare professionals discharging patients are limited. That there is no separate unit for home healthcare service for the follow-up of patients with advanced heart failure is one of the conditions weakening the self-care process.

4.1.3.3 Limited access to healthcare services

In addition to the diagnosis of advanced heart failure, elderly patients who live alone or far from the hospital and have financial problems experience difficulties in accessing healthcare services.

4.2 Self-care evaluation

Heart failure self-care is defined as the process of healthcare and disease management in which the stability of decisions and behaviours is maintained, defined by changes in the patient's condition and for which correct applications are provided. Studies in the field of heart failure have shown the need for healthy lifestyle behaviours, the follow-up and management of symptoms, and determination of the level at which the patient can take responsibility, in addition to treatment compliance.

The international scales used for heart failure patients include the Self-Care of Heart Failure Index, the European Heart Failure Self-Care Behaviour Scale, and the Minnesota Living with Heart Failure Questionnaire [MLWHFQ].

The Self-Care of Heart Failure Index [SCHFI], which is the most comprehensive evaluation scale, has been translated into 22 languages and has been modified several times over the years in accordance with evidence-based practices. The SCHFI version 7.2 consists of four sections of self-care [10 items], symptom perception [11 items], self-care management [8 items], and self-belief [10 items] [22].

The European Heart Failure Self-Care Behaviour Scale is a short self-reported scale of 9 items. The questionnaire includes items related to self-care behaviours of heart failure, consisting of questions directly measuring behaviours associated with fluid and weight management [23].

The Minnesota Living with Heart Failure Questionnaire [MLWHFQ] is a quality of life questionnaire comprising two dimensions [physical and emotional subdimensions] and 21 patient-specific questions. It was designed to measure the effect on the quality of life of heart failure and the treatment received. To date, the questionnaire has been translated into 33 languages, and validity and reliability studies have been conducted [24].

4.3 Self-care behaviours of patients with heart failure

4.3.1 Physical activity

The reduced exercise capacity of patients with advanced stage heart failure is associated with impairments in cardiac and pulmonary reserves, and reduced peripheral and respiratory skeletal muscle perfusion and/or function. Shortness of breath and/or fatigue symptoms in particular cause a decrease in physical activity capacity [25]. In patients with advanced stage heart failure, correct evaluation of the patient's exercise intolerance is an important subject both in the gaining of self-care behaviours and in the determination of medical and device treatment.

Exercise intolerance in advanced stage heart failure is evaluated subjectively in the New York Heart Association [NYHA] functional classification and with health-related quality of life questionnaires. Exercise capacity can be evaluated with objective quantitative methods using the 6-minute walk test [6MWT] and with the cardiopulmonary exercise test [CPX] and graded exercise test with electrocardiography [ECG].

From the subjective methods, the Barthel daily living activities test is a test that can be applied and easily understood by both patients and carers.

Healthcare personnel usually use the 6MWT to evaluate the daily living activity of patients with advanced stage heart failure. The 6MWT is a simple test in which the patient walks at a self-selected speed for 6 minutes along a 30-metre corridor, and the distance covered is measured. The distance walked is useful in providing information about the grade of disease severity and the efficacy of treatment, and in predicting hospitalisations and mortality in heart failure [26, 27].

The CPX is a strong prognostic marker, especially in advanced stage heart failure, and is used to clinically evaluate the risk of unwanted events and candidacy for transplantation. The CPX variables respond positively to pharmacological, lifestyle, and surgical interventions, thereby making serial CPX necessary for the evaluation of therapeutic efficacy [28, 29].

Exercise-based cardiac rehabilitation is a first-class recommendation in the American Heart Association. Medicare and Medicaid Services Centres and most insurance companies in the USA allow for at least 6 weeks [generally 36 sessions] of exercise-based cardiac rehabilitation service for patients with stable chronic heart failure of LVEF <35% and those who despite this have NYHA functional class II and IV symptoms [30].

4.3.2 Pain control

In patients with advanced stage heart failure, monitoring of fluctuations in body weight is a very important self-care behaviour as it can be a sign of an increase in retention of body fluids.

4.3.3 Diet

Cachexia in patients with advanced stage heart failure is associated with a poor prognosis, as it is related to obstruction, inflammation, malabsorption, anorexia, and neurohormonal over-activation. Approximately 5–15% of patients with heart failure experience unwanted weight loss due to reduced skeletal muscle mass, with or without fat tissue depletion [13]. The occurrence of unintended weight loss without oedema of up to >5% within 5–7 months or > 6.12%, or BMI <20 kg/m^2, is defined as cachexia. Therefore, dietary and nutritional evaluation of patients with advanced stage heart failure is important.

In the evaluation of the nutritional status of patients with advanced stage heart failure by healthcare professionals, structured nutritional evaluation tests such as the Subjective Global Assessment [SGA], the Nutritional Risk Screening [NRS] 2002, or the Mini-Nutritional Evaluation are used in addition to analytical and anthropometric parameters. In recent years, the frequently used NRS has been used as a malnutrition-screening tool based on the self-report of the patient and includes items to evaluate the current nutritional status and disease severity [31].

In advanced heart failure, the body passes from an anabolic to a catabolic status with an increase in the levels and activity of catabolic mediators such as pro-inflammatory cytokines and glucocorticoids, and a decrease in the levels and activity of anabolic mediators such as insulin and growth hormone. The increase in protein destruction causes muscle loss [32]. Therefore, the daily calorie and protein intake of patients should be regulated.

4.3.4 Oedema follow-up

Increased activation of the renin-angiotensin-aldosterone system [RAAS] together with increased vasopressin causes a worsening of sodium and fluid retention in patients with advanced heart failure. Pleural effusion and anasarca oedema associated with a volume increase can be seen in patients with advanced heart failure [11].

Oedema becomes evident with an increase of at least 3–5 kg. It is generally bilateral, progresses upwards from the feet as it is mainly determined by gravity, and may form in the trunk, face, and arms. This status can be accompanied by ascites, and pleural and pericardial effusion [33]. Although there is no objective measurement in the classification of oedema, a visual analogue scale and pictures showing the localisation of oedema are generally used in the self-care of patients [34].

Healthcare professionals grade oedema from 1+ to 4+. A grade of 1+ indicates mild oedema in both feet and ankles; 2+ indicates oedema in both feet, legs, and the hands or forearms; 3+ indicates oedema in both lower and upper extremities and in an area of the face region, and 4+ indicates anasarca oedema.

4.3.5 Alcohol consumption and smoking

Excessive alcohol consumption is one of the most important causes of dilated cardiomyopathy [defined as alcoholic cardiomyopathy-ACM], and it is estimated that 40% of dilated cardiomyopathy can be associated with excessive alcohol consumption. This supports that there should be lower alcohol consumption limits than are recommended in many guidelines and that patients with cardiac myopathy should stop drinking to prevent cardiac failure [35].

Nicotine and carbon monoxide in cigarettes are the primary harmful substances in respect of the heart and vascular system. Nicotine increases the pulse rate and the oxygen requirement of the heart, temporarily increases blood pressure, increases blood clotting, and causes atherosclerosis by damaging the endothelial layer. By combining with haemoglobin, carbon monoxide converts to carboxyhaemoglobin, thereby reducing the oxygen transport capacity of the blood and the amount of oxygen going to the tissues.

4.3.6 Sleep

Patients with advanced stage heart failure often experience insufficient and poor-quality sleep because of periods of pulmonary fluid overloading, resulting in orthopnoea, paroxysmal nocturnal dyspnoea, and nocturia [36].

Respiratory disorders during sleep affect >50% of patients with low ejection fraction. When heart failure becomes more severe, there is an evident increase in the prevalence of Cheyne-Stokes respiration with central sleep apnoea [characterised by a ventilation pattern expressed with hypocapnia associated with hyperventilation]. Another main type of sleep disorder often seen in heart failure patients is obstructive sleep apnoea [OSA]. OSA is especially common if the patient is overweight, has diabetes, and has a large neck circumference, or if there is retro or prognathism. In addition, OSA is accepted as one of the comorbidities contributing to low ejection fraction.

The determination and recording of factors affecting sleep, such as changes in sleep and activity, diet, and drugs used, is important for the provision of sleep hygiene.

4.3.7 Compliance with drugs and treatment

According to the recommendations of the ESC/HFA guidelines related to heart failure, regular follow-up and monitoring of biomedical parameters is useful in providing safety and the optimal dose of drugs and the determination of the development of complications or disease progression [37].

Pharmacological treatment of heart failure consists of several different drugs that have different dose strategies, especially in heart failure patients with reduced ejection fraction [HFrEF]. When the drugs for frequently seen comorbidities such as atrial fibrillation, hypertension, and diabetes are taken into consideration, the result is a labyrinthine, continuously changing drug regimen that requires time, presence of mind, and dedication for successful compliance [38].

4.3.8 Symptom perception

Symptom perception is related to signs observed and listening to the body to determine physical sensations allowing the patient to identify, interpret, and label symptoms. Symptom awareness, with measurement and taking rapid action through evaluation, is defined as one of the basic elements in the self-care process of patients with advanced heart failure [39].

Symptom evaluation by the patient is assessed under the headings of frequency, intensity [e.g., on a scale of 1–10], rate [how many times in a time interval], duration, model [mornings, after activity, etc.], symptom specificity [in the whole body, in the arms, etc.], and pain [20]. In addition to clinical evaluation, symptoms can be evaluated using the Numerical Grading Scale, the Edmonton Symptom Assessment Scale [ESAS], the ESAS-HF, or the Integrated Palliative Care Outcome Scale.

4.3.9 Cognitive status

Heart failure causes neurohormonal, inflammatory, and hemodynamic abnormalities, which are thought to contribute to all cognitive disorders. There is at least a mild-level cognitive disorder in approximately 70% of patients with heart failure, and this has been shown to be associated with poor self-care.

4.4 The monitoring of self-care in patients with advanced heart failure

The monitoring of self-care behaviours is a data collection tool. The European Cardiology Association guidelines recommend regular follow-up of heart failure patients by healthcare providers. Symptom monitoring can be supported by distant follow-up or the personal monitoring by family members, unofficial carers, and healthcare specialists. The importance of vital findings and symptoms in patients with advanced heart failure has been stated in all the guidelines. The methods that can be useful in the monitoring of symptoms by the patients themselves and by healthcare professionals can be grouped as mHealth Tools and paper-based tools to determine the signs of heart failure, and medical devices and tools consulted by healthcare specialists to determine the signs of heart failure [40].

4.4.1 mHealth tools to determine the signs of advanced heart failure

4.4.1.1 Smartphone applications

Smartphone applications can be used to measure blood sugar levels and blood pressure, heart rate, and even blood oxygen fullness, and to monitor sleep, stress levels, and the activities of patients with advanced heart failure. In the light of the patient information evaluated, smartphone applications can be used as a retrospective record store with the related records of the patient status [41]. In addition, it can function as a reminder of drugs taken at previously defined times and as a list of symptoms, signs and drugs when the status of the patient worsened.

4.4.2 Paper-based tools to determine the signs of advanced heart failure

Daily: the daily use of these to support self-care, especially at home, is a daily record of weight, vital signs, nutrition, water and salt consumption, drugs used, symptoms seen, and fear and concerns of the patient and can be a very important data source for healthcare professionals, providing information independently of the self-care of the patient.

Brochure with Schematic Warning Signs: these are used by patients marking on brochures showing the form of symptoms of heart failure.

4.4.3 Medical devices determining the signs of advanced heart failure

To monitor the bodily fluid retention of patients, scales and the Vest to Measure Pulmonary Fluid can be used.

4.4.4 Tools consulted by healthcare professionals to determine the signs of advanced heart failure

Visual video consultations can provide savings in time, energy, and hospital resources. A telephone number on which healthcare professionals can be directly contacted is important for early intervention to symptoms of patients with advanced heart failure [42].

4.5 The management of self-care behaviours of patients with advanced heart failure

The management of self-care is the process of decision-making and appropriate response for the patient to appropriately manage functions related to him/herself. Self-care management of patients with advanced heart failure is defined as taking responsibility for the management of disease-related symptoms, treatment, and maintaining healthy lifestyle behaviours. Self-care management is provided by the patient, the primary carer, and healthcare professionals.

The self-care management of patients with advanced stage heart failure is formed of the stages of knowledge, awareness, determination, decision-making, and application.

4.5.1 Evaluation of self-care management

Following the definition of the concept of the self-care management process [SCMP] by Jones and Preuett, the SCMP was developed with testing [43], and the characteristics of the concept were protected with explanations and additions [44].

4.5.2 Management of physical activity

Lifestyle exercises [walking, using stairs when possible, parking at a distance from shops, light gardening, and dancing] and structured activities and exercise can be useful as a priority for patients with heart failure. However, especially in patients with advanced heart failure, supervised exercise is recommended to increase exercise tolerance and improve quality of life [30]. One of the aims of self-care behaviours is for patients with advanced stage heart failure to come to a condition in which gradual mobilisation or stretching/relaxing movements of small muscle groups can be made and daily living activities can be performed.

4.5.3 Drug management

Different pharmacological combinations are used in the treatment of advanced heart failure. The aim in self-care management is to provide drug compliance of the patient. Within drug compliance, the patient is expected to adhere to the principles of rational drug use. These principles are that drugs are taken at the prescribed time and dose, that the patient has information about the drugs, and that vital signs and drug-related symptoms are recorded and healthcare professionals are informed. In recent years, many interventions have been developed to increase the drug compliance of cardiovascular disease patients, including technical interventions such as drug reminder applications, educational interventions, and interventions to increase motivation.

4.5.4 Oedema control, water and salt restrictions

The control of fluid intake is the primary nutritional recommendation. Daily fluid intake should be at the level of 1500–2000 ml, and daily weight follow-up should be made in respect of rapid weight increases. Salt restriction is a lifestyle change that should not be neglected in heart failure patients. In the American Heart Society guidelines, salt consumption of <3gr/day is recommended for symptomatic grade C and D patients [43]. The education of patients and their carers in respect of water and sodium restrictions and their follow-up are extremely important. Sodium-restricted diets can reduce total calorie and/or macro- and micronutrient intake and can therefore worsen the nutritional status [44].

4.5.5 Diet

Daily energy intake should be 25–30 Kcal/kg/day, and the amount of protein intake should be 1.5–2 gr/kg/day. Cholesterol in the diet should be restricted to be <200 mg per day; more foods containing unsaturated fat should be given, and fatty dairy products and foods high in saturated fats should be avoided [43].

The frequent use of diuretics leads to a decrease in potassium, sodium, and magnesium levels, and an increase in uric acid, blood glucose, and lipids. Those taking diuretics that lose potassium can be recommended to consume more foods with a high potassium content such as prunes, bananas, apricots, soya, oranges, broccoli, melon, tomatoes, spinach, and potatoes. Recommended herbal products include daily 1–2 cloves of garlic, 200–300 mg hawthorn extract, 1500 mg calcium, and 500 mg magnesium supplements. Thiamin, selenium, magnesium, zinc, calcium, and vitamin D deficiencies are frequently seen in patients with heart failure. It has been shown that with the addition of micronutrients such as iron, copper, selenium, riboflavin, folate, and vitamins A, B1, B6, B12, C, D, and E to the treatment of these patients, exercise tolerance has increased and symptoms have decreased [42]. When oral nutrition remains insufficient, enteral nutrition can be applied with foods high in protein concentration. This can be changed to parenteral feeding when the gastrointestinal system is significantly affected [45].

4.5.6 Sleep management

In cases with heart failure and obstructive sleep apnoea [OSA], positive pressure mask treatment [CPAP] can be considered. There is some evidence that OSA symptoms, cardiac function, biomarkers of cardiovascular disease, and quality of life can improve with CPAP treatment in patients with heart failure, but there is little evidence of an improvement in mortality [36].

As there can be a higher mortality rate in patients with predominantly central sleep apnoea and low ejection fraction, they should be applied with adaptive servo-ventilation.

4.5.7 Symptom management

It is important to convert to behaviour the teaching given by healthcare professionals of advanced heart failure symptoms and observe progression, symptom identification, support for listening to the body, and/or interpretation of heart failure symptoms. Follow-up of patient behaviours must be performed by healthcare professionals. Follow-up should be made with a symptom diary kept by the patient, heart failure decompensation, and criteria for hospitalisation and mortality [39].

4.5.8 Breathing exercises

Advanced stage heart failure causes a decrease in cardiac flow and in the blood flow of peripheral and respiratory muscles. These changes can cause muscle dysfunction leading to fibre atrophy [basically type I] and weakness in peripheral and respiratory muscles. Therefore, muscle weakness related to frequent shortness of breath can cause fatigue, reduced functional capacity, and increased exercise intolerance in these patients. In this context, inspiratory muscle training [IMT] can be used as an assistive intervention to develop cardiopulmonary capacity in these individuals. Strengthening of the respiratory muscles provides more efficient airway clearance, inspiratory pressure, and maximal expiration, and prevents fatigue of the respiratory muscles [46].

Breathing exercises regulate cardiac parameters such as respiration, ejection fraction, aortic pressure, pulmonary artery pressure, and tissue oxygenation [47]. Slow breathing exercises are defined according to a controlled respiratory rate to reduce respiratory rate and increase respiratory breadth [tidal volume].

Deep breathing exercises are a form of exercise that focus on deep and slow respiration at targeted breaths per minute using the diaphragm.

4.5.9 Preventing falls

In parallel with existing symptoms and the age of patients with advanced heart failure, evaluations of the risk of falling, drug-related risks, exercise capacity, and walking and balance are included in the clinical practice guidelines of risk management [48].

4.5.10 Psychosocial support

There has been increasing interest in the use of stress management interventions, including mindfulness-based interventions [MBIs], for the alleviation of psychological problems and the improvement of physical health outcomes [49].

4.5.11 Protection against infection

Vaccination against influenza and pneumococcal infections is recommended by the European Society of Cardiology. Unless there are contraindications, it is recommended that heart failure patients are vaccinated against influenza every year and against pneumococcal infections once every 5 years.

Self-care in heart failure patients is very important for the improvement of patient outcomes, including quality of life, and lower hospitalisation and mortality rates. In this chapter, the information has been reviewed related to the factors affecting the self-care of patients with advanced stage heart failure, the behaviours necessary for self-care [how diet can be adhered to, which symptoms are to be monitored], and how self-care can be managed and monitored. Symptom management and treatment compliance behaviours in patients with advanced heart failure are the most important self-care behaviours that affect the patient's quality of life and survival, and it is not possible for these behaviours to be managed only by the patient and their relatives. The biggest risk for patients and their relatives is that they may not even be aware of the incomplete/incorrect information or practices in the self-care behaviours they learn and apply. Collaboration of multidisciplinary health professionals such as physicians, nurses, psychologists, and dietitians who are autonomous in the field of heart failure is the golden criterion in the management of the advanced stage heart failure self-care process. Autonomous healthcare professionals in the field of heart failure know what needs to happen before taking action on issues related to their patient; notice what is not; perceive, interpret, and associate new situations; and ensure that the process progresses positively by directing and monitoring the patient to the right team member in a timely manner.

Author details

Füsun Afşar
Maltepe University School of Nursing, Istanbul, Türkiye

*Address all correspondence to: fusunafsar@maltepe.edut.r

References

[1] Massouh A, Skouri H, Cook P, Huijer HAS, Khoury M, Meek P. Self-care confidence mediates self-care maintenance and management in patients with heart failure. Heart & Lung. 2020;**49**(1):30-35. DOI: 10.1016/j.hrtlng.2019.07.008

[2] McHorney CA, Mansukhani SG, Anatchkova M, Taylor N, Wirtz HS, Abbasi S, et al. The impact of heart failure on patients and caregivers: A qualitative study. PLoS One. 2021;**16**(3):e0248240. DOI: 10.1371/journal.pone.0248240

[3] Negarandeh R, Aghajanloo A, Seylani K. Barriers to self-care among patients with heart failure: A qualitative study. Journal of Caring Sciences. 2020;**10**(4):196-204. DOI: 10.34172/jcs.2020.026

[4] King KC, Goldstein S. Congestive heart failure and pulmonary Edema. In: StatPearls [Internet]. Treasure Island [FL]: StatPearls Publishing; 2023. Available from: https://www.ncbi.nlm.nih.gov/books/NBK554557/

[5] Saha S. Self-care Education for Heart Failure Patient. Degree Thesis in Health Care and Social Welfare. Vaasa: NOVIA University of Applied Sciences; 2022

[6] Tomasoni D, Vishram-Nielsen JKK, Pagnesi M, Adamo M, Lombardi CM, Gustafsson F, et al. Advanced heart failure: Guideline-directed medical therapy, diuretics, inotropes, and palliative care. ESC Heart Failure. 2022;**9**(3):1507-1523. DOI: 10.1002/ehf2.13859

[7] Truby LK, Rogers JG. Advanced heart failure: Epidemiology, diagnosis, and therapeutic approaches. JACC: Heart Failure. 2020;**8**(7):523-536. DOI: 10.1016/j.jchf.2020.01.014

[8] Nalbantgil S, Çavuşoğlu Y, Akdeniz B, Altay H, Çelik A, Engin Ç, et al. Guide on advanced heart failure. Updates in Cardiology. 2018;**1**(1):1-79. DOI: 10.5543/ucard.2018.43153

[9] Bozkurt B, Coats AJS, Tsutsui H, Abdelhamid CM, Adamopoulos S, Albert N, et al. European Journal of Heart Failure. 2021;**23**(3):352-380. DOI: 10.1002/ejhf.2115 Epub 2021 Mar 3

[10] Jurgens CY, Lee CS, Aycock DM, Masterson Creber R, Denfeld QE, DeVon HA, et al. A scientific statement from the American Heart Association. Circulation. 2022;**146**:e173-e184. DOI: 10.1161/CIR.0000000000001089

[11] Yıldız Ayvaz M, Enç N. Edema in heart failure. Turkish Journal of Cardiovascular Nursing. 2018;**9**(19):69-75. DOI: 10.5543/khd.2018.14632

[12] Lee JH, Hwang KK. End-of-life Care for end-stage Heart Failure Patients. Korean Circulation Journal. 2022;**52**(9):659-679. DOI: 10.4070/kcj.2022.0211

[13] McDonagh TA, Metra M, Adamo M, Gardner RS, Baumbach A, Böhm M, et al. 2021 ESC guidelines for the diagnosis and treatment of acute and chronic heart failure: Developed by the task force for the diagnosis and treatment of acute and chronic heart failure of the European Society of Cardiology [ESC]. With the special contribution of the heart failure association [HFA] of the ESC. European Journal of Heart Failure. 2022;**24**(1):4-131. DOI: 10.1002/ejhf.2333

[14] Avcı A, Gün M. Sleep problems in patients with heart failure and non-pharmacological treatment. Turkish Journal of Cardiovascular Nursing.

2020;**11**(25):90-99. DOI: 10.5543/khd.2020.30974

[15] Arzt M, Oldenburg O, Graml A, Schnepf J, Erdmann E, Teschler H, et al. Prevalence and predictors of sleep-disordered breathing in chronic heart failure: The SchlaHF-XT registry. ESC Heart Failure. 2022;**9**(6):4100-4111. DOI: 10.1002/ehf2.14027

[16] Hsu MY, Chiang CW, Chiou AF. The effects of a self-regulation programme on self-care behaviour in patients with heart failure: A randomized controlled trial. International Journal of Nursing Studies. 2021;**116**:103778. DOI: 10.1016/j.ijnurstu.2020.103778

[17] WHO guideline on self-care interventions for health and well-being. 2022 [revision: Executive summary] [9789240030909-eng.pdf] [Accessed: August 01, 2023]

[18] Lee KS, Choi JO, Jeon ES, Park JH, Jung MS, Lee Z, et al. Distinct factors associated with better self-care in heart failure patients with and without mild cognitive impairment. The Journal of Cardiovascular Nursing. 2019;**34**(6):440-447. DOI: 10.1097/JCN.0000000000000600

[19] Riegel B, Dickson VV, Vellone E. The situation-specific theory of heart failure self-care: An update on the problem, person, and environmental factors influencing heart failure self-care. The Journal of Cardiovascular Nursing. 2022;**37**(6):515-529. DOI: 10.1097/JCN.0000000000000919

[20] Jaarsma T, Hill L, Bayes-Genis A, La Rocca HB, Castiello T, Čelutkienė J, et al. Self-care of heart failure patients: Practical management recommendations from the heart failure Association of the European Society of cardiology. European Journal of Heart Failure. 2021;**23**(1):157-174. DOI: 10.1002/ejhf.2008

[21] Liljeroos M, Kato NP, van der Wal MH, Brons M, Luttik ML, van Veldhuisen DJ, et al. Trajectory of self-care behaviour in patients with heart failure: The impact on clinical outcomes and influencing factors. European Journal of Cardiovascular Nursing. 2020;**19**(5):421-432. DOI: 10.1177/1474515120902317

[22] Vellone E, Maria M, Iovino P, Barbaranelli C, Zeffiro V, Pucciarelli G, et al. The self-care of heart failure index version 7.2: Further psychometric testing. Research in Nursing & Health. 2020;**43**(6):640-650. DOI: 10.1002/nur.22083

[23] Jaarsma T, Strömberg A, Mårtensson J, Dracup K. Development and testing of the European heart failure self-care behaviour scale. European Journal of Heart Failure. 2003;**5**(3):363-370. DOI: 10.1016/s1388-9842[02]00253-2

[24] Rector TS, Cohn JN. Assessment of patient outcome with the Minnesota living with heart failure questionnaire: Reliability and validity during a randomized, double-blind, placebo-controlled trial of pimobendan. Pimobendan Multicenter research group. American Heart Journal. 1992;**124**(4):1017-1025. DOI: 10.1016/0002-8703[92]90986-6

[25] Nijholt KT, Sánchez-Aguilera PI, Voorrips SN, de Boer RA, Westenbrink BD. Exercise: A molecular tool to boost muscle growth and mitochondrial performance in heart failure? European Journal of Heart Failure. 2022;**24**(2):287-298. DOI: 10.1002/ejhf.2407

[26] Nayor M, Houstis NE, Namasivayam M, Rouvina J, Hardin C,

Shah RV, et al. Impaired exercise tolerance in heart failure with preserved ejection fraction: Quantification of multiorgan system reserve capacity. JACC Heart Failure. 2020;**8**(8):605-617. DOI: 10.1016/j.jchf.2020.03.008

[27] Crisci G, De Luca M, D'Assante R, Ranieri B, D'Agostino A, Valente V, et al. Effects of exercise on heart failure with preserved ejection fraction: An updated review of literature. Journal of Cardiovascular Development and Disease. 2022;**9**(8):241. DOI: 10.3390/jcdd9080241

[28] Del Buono MG, Arena R, Borlaug BA, Carbone S, Canada JM, Kirkman DL, et al. Exercise intolerance in patients with heart failure: JACC state-of-the-art review. Journal of the American College of Cardiology. 2019;**73**(17):2209-2225. DOI: 10.1016/j.jacc.2019.01.072

[29] Giannitsi S, Bougiakli M, Bechlioulis A, Kotsia A, Michalis LK, Naka KK. 6-minute walking test: A useful tool in the management of heart failure patients. Therapeutic Advances in Cardiovascular Disease. 2019;**13**:1753944719870084. DOI: 10.1177/1753944719870084

[30] Bozkurt B, Fonarow GC, Goldberg LR, Guglin M, Josephson RA, Forman DE, et al. ACC's heart failure and transplant section and leadership council. Cardiac rehabilitation for patients with heart failure: JACC expert panel. Journal of the American College of Cardiology. 2021;**77**(11):1454-1469. DOI: 10.1016/j.jacc.2021.01.030

[31] Hersberger L, Dietz A, Bürgler H, Bargetzi A, Bargetzi L, Kägi-Braun N, et al. Individualized nutritional support for hospitalized patients with chronic heart failure. Journal of the American College of Cardiology. 2021;**77**(18):2307-2319. DOI: 10.1016/j.jacc.2021.03.232

[32] Habaybeh D, de Moraes MB, Slee A, Avgerinou C. Nutritional interventions for heart failure patients who are malnourished or at risk of malnutrition or cachexia: A systematic review and meta-analysis. Heart Failure Reviews. 2021;**26**(5):1103-1118. DOI: 10.1007/s10741-020-09937-9

[33] Koshy AO, Gallivan ER, McGinlay M, Straw S, Drozd M, Toms AG, et al. Prioritizing symptom management in the treatment of chronic heart failure. ESC Heart Failure. 2020;**7**(5):2193-2207. DOI: 10.1002/ehf2.12875

[34] Salyer J, Flattery M, Lyon DE. Heart failure symptom clusters and quality of life. Heart & Lung. 2019;**48**(5):366-372. DOI: 10.1016/j.hrtlng.2019.05.016

[35] Piepoli MF, Adamo M, Barison A, Bestetti RB, Biegus J, Böhm M, et al. Preventing heart failure: A position paper of the heart failure association in collaboration with the European Association of Preventive Cardiology. European Journal of Preventive Cardiology. 2022;**29**(1):275-300. DOI: 10.1093/eurjpc/zwab147

[36] Yeghiazarians Y, Jneid H, Tietjens JR, Redline S, Brown DL, El-Sherif N, et al. Obstructive sleep Apnea and cardiovascular disease: A scientific statement from the American Heart Association. Circulation. 2021;**144**(3):e56-e67. DOI: 10.1161/CIR.0000000000000988

[37] Rosano GMC, Vitale C, Adamo M, Metra M. Roadmap for the management of heart failure patients during the vulnerable phase after heart failure hospitalizations: How to implement excellence in clinical practice. Journal of Cardiovascular Medicine [Hagerstown]. 2022;**23**(3):149-156. DOI: 10.2459/JCM.0000000000001221

[38] Bakogiannis C, Tsarouchas A, Mouselimis D, Lazaridis C, Theofillogianakos EK, Billis A, et al. A patient-oriented app [ThessHF] to improve self-care quality in heart failure: From evidence-based design to pilot study. JMIR mHealth and uHealth. 2021;**9**(4):e24271. DOI: 10.2196/24271

[39] Santos GC, Liljeroos M, Dwyer AA, Jaques C, Girard J, Strömberg A, et al. Symptom perception in heart failure - interventions and outcomes: A scoping review. International Journal of Nursing Studies. 2021;**116**:103524. DOI: 10.1016/j.ijnurstu.2020.103524

[40] Atherton JJ, Sindone A, de Pasquale CG, Driscoll A, PS MD, Hopper I, et al. Guidelines for the prevention, detection, and management of heart failure in Australia. Heart, Lung & Circulation. 2018;**27**(10):1123-1208. DOI: 10.1016/j.hlc.2018.06.1042

[41] Leclercq C, Witt H, Hindricks G, Katra RP, Albert D, Belliger A, et al. Wearables, telemedicine, and artificial intelligence in arrhythmias and heart failure: Proceedings of the European Society of Cardiology Cardiovascular Round Table. Europace. 2022;**24**(9):1372-1383. DOI: 10.1093/europace/euac052

[42] Indraratna P, Biswas U, McVeigh J, Mamo A, Magdy J, Vickers D, et al. Smartphone-based model of care to support patients with cardiac disease transitioning from hospital to the community [TeleClinical care]: Pilot randomized controlled trial. JMIR mHealth and uHealth. 2022;**10**(2):e32554. DOI: 10.2196/32554

[43] Kida K, Miyajima I, Suzuki N, Greenberg BH, Akashi YJ. Nutritional management of heart failure. Journal of Cardiology. 2023;**81**:283-291. DOI: 10.1016/j.jjcg.2022.11.001

[44] Billingsley HE, Hummel SL, Carbone S. The role of diet and nutrition in heart failure: A state-of-the-art narrative review. Progress in Cardiovascular Diseases. 2020;**63**(5):538-551. DOI: 10.1016/j.pcad.2020.08.004

[45] Güler MS, Fedai H, Demirbağ R. Healthy nutrition recommendations in cardiovascular diseases. Journal of Harran University Medical Faculty. 2021;**18**(2):342-348. DOI: 10.35440/hutfd.947849

[46] Çaylan K, Otağ A. Breath exercises and effective exercise therapies in heart failure. Turkish Journal of Science and Health. 2020;**1**(2):84-93 ISSN: 2717-7173

[47] Janardan C, Madhavi K. Influence of music therapy and breathıng exercises on anxiety ın post-operatıve cardiac dıseased individuals. International Journal of Physiotherapy. 2016;**3**(1):22-28. DOI: 10.15621/IJPHY/2016/V3I1/88903

[48] Montero-Odasso MM, Kamkar N, Pieruccini-Faria F, Osman A, Sarquis-Adamson Y, Close J, et al. Task force on global guidelines for falls in older adults. Evaluation of clinical practice guidelines on fall prevention and Management for Older Adults: A systematic review. JAMA Network Open. 2021;**4**(12):e2138911. DOI: 10.1001/jamanetworkopen.2021.38911

[49] Scott-Sheldon LAJ, Gathright EC, Donahue ML, Balletto B, Feulner MM, DeCosta J, et al. Mindfulness-based interventions for adults with cardiovascular disease: A systematic review and meta-analysis. Annals of Behavioral Medicine. 2020;**54**(1):67-73. DOI: 10.1093/abm/kaz020

Chapter 2

Cardiac Reshaping Net for Dilated Cardiomyopathy

Toshiaki Akita, Sho Akita, Hideki Ito, Masato Mutsuga and Toshiya Sasaki

Abstract

Dilated cardiomyopathy (DCM) is an intractable disease that progressively worsens with cardiac enlargement and heart failure. There are approximately 20,000 patients designated with intractable disease who have moderate or severe heart failure symptoms even with appropriate medical treatment, making it the most common target disease for heart transplantation in Japan. Sixty percent of designated DCM patients are over the age of 60. If we can extend their healthy life expectancy by 5 to 10 years, we can reduce the number of patients who are candidates for heart transplantation. We have developed a patient-specific cardiac reshaping net (PS-CRN) to prevent progressive cardiac enlargement (=cardiac remodeling), which is the major factor in worsening heart failure. We have conducted three first-in-human clinical trials. The past and present of the "cardiac support net therapy" will be reviewed.

Keywords: dilated cardiomyopathy, cardiac remodeling, cardiac remodeling, heart failure with reduced ejection fraction (HFrEF), left ventricular end-diastolic pressure-volume relationship, right ventricular diastolic function, functional mitral regurgitation, precision medicine

1. Introduction

1.1 General treatment of advanced heart failure

The number of heart failure patients is rapidly increasing worldwide, creating a heart failure pandemic. Heart transplantation is the only radical treatment for patients with end-stage heart failure, but the shortage of donors severely limits its use. Although survival rates with continuous-flow ventricular assist devices have improved dramatically in recent years, they are not widely available because they are extremely expensive, require significant medical resources, and are associated with a high rate of serious complications. Effective and widely available treatments are urgently needed.

1.2 Dilated cardiomyopathy and cardiac remodeling

Regardless of the underlying disease, heart failure is further compromised by progressive enlargement of the heart. The decline in cardiac function and the progressive enlargement of the heart are linked, a phenomenon known as cardiac remodeling. Cardiac remodeling, after myocardial infarction, correlates with worse life outcomes, and prevention of cardiac remodeling has become a therapeutic goal [1].

1.3 Problems with previous cardiac support net therapy (Acorn CorCap, Paracor)

Devices to prevent cardiac remodeling by physical means, such as covering the ventricles with polyester mesh bags (Acorn CorCap) or shape memory alloy (Paracor), have been developed and used in humans since about 2000 [2–5].

The Acorn CorCap is the most extensively studied of these devices and received CE mark approval in 2001. Randomized clinical trials of 300 cases have been performed in the United States [2, 3, 6, 7]. Although it demonstrated reverse cardiac remodeling, it did not demonstrate prognostic value and was not approved by the FDA. There was a lot of missing data on the primary endpoint (NYHA), and Acorn Cardiovascular, the company developing the device, did not comply with the FDA's request for corrections. On the other hand, the FDA reviewers agreed with the need for this type of device.

The Acorn CorCap wraps the right and left ventricles equally, so applying the necessary pressure (>5 mmHg) to the left ventricle would impair right ventricular dilation and reduce cardiac output (**Figure 1** left panel) [8, 9]. At a contact pressure of 3 mmHg or higher on the ventricle, transmural myocardial pressure (Ptm) decreased in the left ventricle, while no change occurred in the right ventricle. At pressures of 5 mmHg or higher, RVEDP and CVP increased, and mean blood pressure decreased [9]. On the other hand, in the device that pressurized only the left ventricle, there

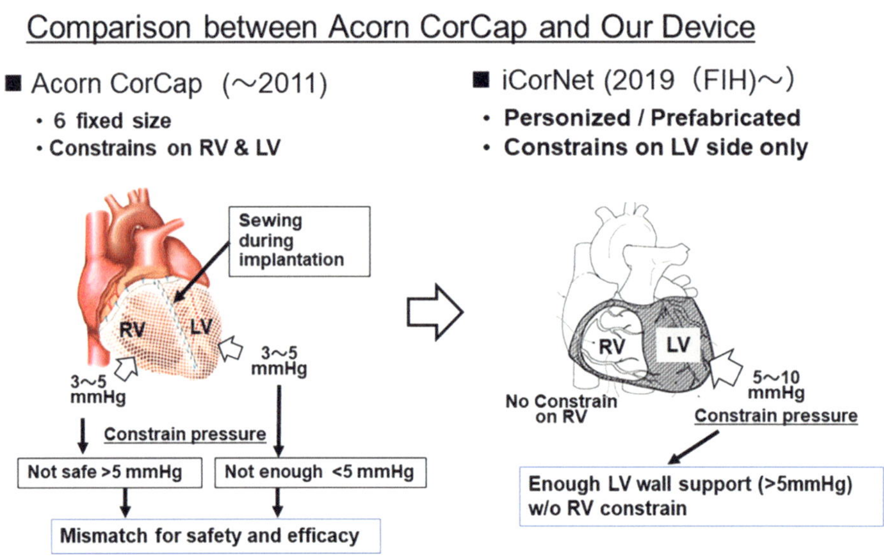

Figure 1.
Comparison between Acorn CorCap and our device. (Left panel) Acorn CorCap has six sizes. The surgeon had to adjust the size to fit. Acorn described that the contact pressure should be 3-5 mmHg. More than 5 mmHg contact pressure on the right ventricular side depresses right ventricular diastolic function. Less than 5 mmHg on the left ventricular side is not sufficient to achieve a meaningful improvement in left ventricular systolic function. (Right panel) iCorNet patient-specific cardiac reshaping net with a hole on the right ventricular side. It is a personalized/prefabricated product that constrains only on the LV side. It can provide sufficient LV wall support (>5 mmHg) without RV constraint.

was no increase in CVP and no decrease in mean blood pressure [8], even when the pressure on the left ventricle was increased up to 14 mmHg. Pressure-volume area and stroke work, which are indirect measures of oxygen consumption, were significantly reduced, and energy efficiency was improved [8].

2. Method and results of experimental study

2.1 Cardiac support net with patient-specific design

In 2005, I read a newspaper article introducing a computer-controlled three-dimensional (3D) knitting machine (Shimaseiki Co. Ltd., Wakayama, Japan). This machine can produce 3D knitted product without sewing "WHOLEGARMENT". I came up with an idea that if we prefabricate patient-specific cardiac support net with this computer-controlled 3D knitting machine using the patient's heart images, then we do not need to adjust the net size (**Figure 1**. right panel). It will eliminate the surgeon's arbitrary adjustment and shorten the operation time.

2.2 Experimental study to determine the suitable size and shape of cardiac support net

In order to eliminate the arbitrary adjustment of the cardiac support net, we need to determine the most appropriate size before the operation. For this purpose, we investigated the systolic and diastolic functions of the right and left ventricles with different sizes of the cardiac support net in a porcine model of chronic heart failure (HF). The HF model was established by rapid atrial pacing (200 bpm for 3 weeks) using a commercial intravenous pacing leadwire and an experimental pacing system (Taishoikakikai Co, Osaka, Japan).

After 3 weeks of rapid pacing, LVDd increased from 34.2 ± 7.0 to 51.0 ± 4.5 mm, and LVDs increased from 24.0 ± 7.1 mm to 46.3 ± 5.2 mm5., respectively. LVEF decreased from 60.6 ± 12.5 to 20.8 ± 8.5% (**Table 1**). We then examined the effects on right and left ventricular pressure-volume relations. The Sigma5 system (CardioDynamics, Zoetermeer, The Netherlands) was used. End-systolic and end-diastolic pressure-volume relations were measured by rapid volume loading with 500 ml of lactated Ringer's solution. The solution was equilibrated with blood before infusion.

We found that the slope of Emax (= end-systolic pressure-volume ratio), which is the most reliable systolic function independent of preload and afterload conditions, became steeper in both right and left ventricles when smaller nets were applied

Atrial Pacing 200 bpm for 3 weeks		
	Before	**After 3 weeks**
LVDd(mm)	34.2 ± 7.0	51.0 ± 4.5
LVDs(mm)	24.0 ± 7.1	46.3 ± 5.2
LVEF(%)	60.6 ± 12.5	20.8 ± 8.5

Table 1.
Change in UCG parameters before and after rapid pacing.

(**Figures** 2 and **3a**: Improvement in Contractility). However, the end-diastolic pressure-volume relation (EDPVR) also shifted to the left and upward, indicating a worsening of diastolic function (**Figures** 2 and **3b**) [10]. The deterioration of the right ventricular diastolic function was more pronounced than that of the left ventricle, especially at 85% of the original heart size (**Figure 3b**). There was a point at which RVEDV stopped increasing in response to rapid volume loading, and from that point only RVEDP increased (**Figure 2b**). This phenomenon was speculated to be due to compression of the right ventricle by the left ventricle and the cardiac support net, which prevented right ventricular dilation. The cardiac support net lowers Ptm, thereby improving left ventricular contractility. However, the positive effect of the cardiac support net on systolic function is offset by the decrease in stroke volume due to the worsening of right ventricular diastolic function [8].

2.3 Patient-specific cardiac reshaping net (PS-CRN) with less constraint on RV side

Based on the above experimental results, we developed a patient-specific cardiac reshaping net (PS-CRN) with less constraint on the right ventricle (RV) by making a hole on the right ventricle side (**Figure 1**) [11]. PS-CRN is made of polyester fiber thread and is prefabricated using computer-controlled knitting machine. The size and shape are designed base on the patient's cardiac images (MRI or contrasted CT) and left ventricular end-diastolic pressure. The relationship between left ventricular end-diastolic pressure and volume is calculated using the Klotz equation [12], The PS-CRN is then designed to achieve 5 to 10 mmHg contact pressure on the LV.

1. The design and manufacturing process is as follows (**Figure 4**)

    i. Cardiac imaging (MRI T2 Whole Heart or Contrast CT).

    ii. Cardiac catheterization: Measurement of LVEDP.

    iii. 3D modeling of LV & RV cavity, whole ventricle surface from cardiac images

    iv. (Converted to STL data).

    v. Create design paper for computer-controlled knitting machine from 3D cardiac model (custom software), setting contact pressure 5 to 10 mmHg on LV surface at LVEDP 30 mmHg).

    vi. Prefabrication of the PS-CRN by computer-controlled knitting machine.

    vii. Washing and packaging with insertion tool and sterilization.

2. What are the important aspects of cardiac assist device therapy?

In heart failure patients, cardiac output decreases above a certain LVEDP point (usually LVEDP >30 mmHg), known as the descending slope of the Frank-Starling curve. Therefore, it is reasonable to set sufficient compression pressure (close to 10 mmHg) above the point of the descending slope of the Frank-Starling curve to

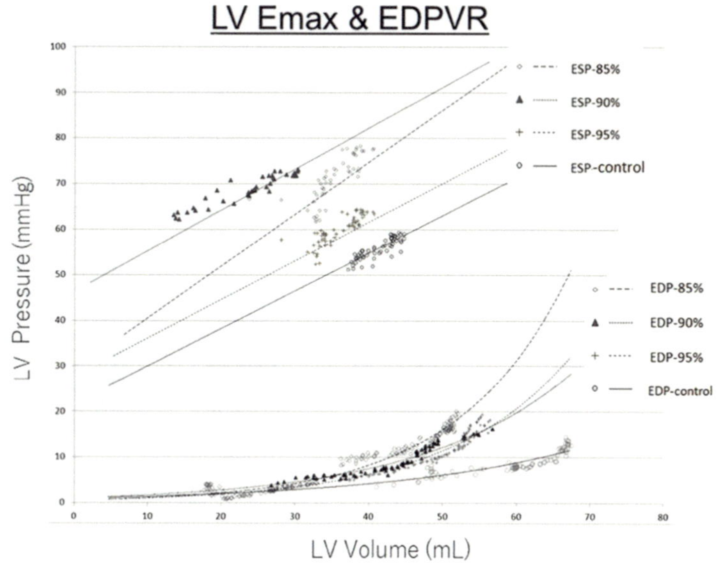

(a)

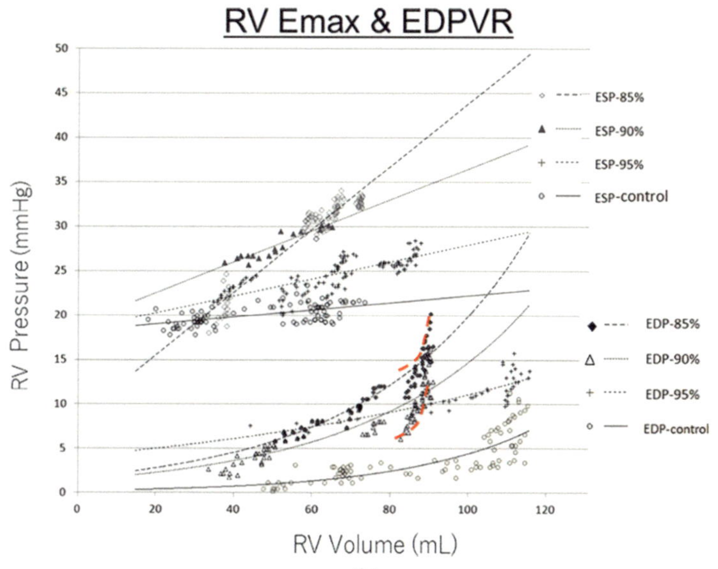

(b)

Figure 2.
a. LV ESPVR & EDPVR. Typical recordings of LV Emax (ESPVR) and EDPVR. Wearing a smaller cardiac net tended to increase Emax. LV EDPVR shifted upward and to the left by wearing a smaller cardiac net. b. RV Emax & EDPVR. Typical recordings of RV Emax (ESPVR) and EDPVR. Wearing a smaller cardiac net tended to increase Emax. RV EDPVR shifted upward and to the left by wearing a smaller cardiac net. Under the 90% size of the cardiac net, RVEDP increased sharply (red dotted line), which meant that RVEDV did not increase further by rapid fluid infusion.

prevent further dilation. This is another important consideration in the design of the PS-CRN in addition to less right ventricular constraint.

The PS-CRN is designed to set the surface pressure on the left ventricular side to 5 to 10 mmHg at LVEDP 30 mmHg. This requires prediction of the LV end-diastolic

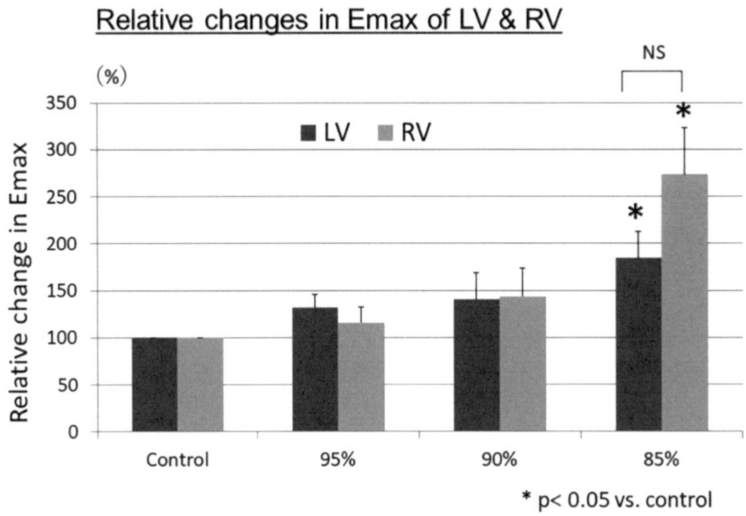

(a)

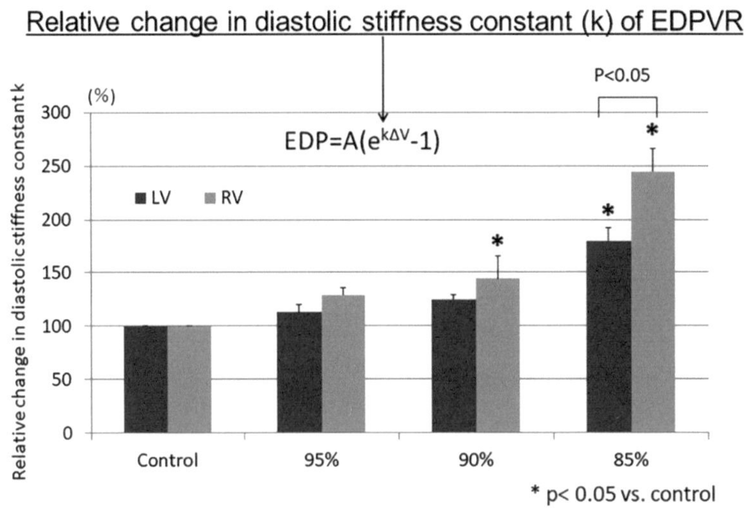

(b)

Figure 3.
a. Relative changes in Emax (end-systolic pressure-volume relation) of LV & RV. The CHF swine model was created by rapid atrial pacing at 200 bpm for 3 weeks. LVEF decreased from 60.6 ± 12.5 to 20.8 ± 8.5% after 3 weeks of rapid pacing. Conductance and pressure catheters were placed in both ventricles and pressure and volume were recorded using the Sigma5 system. A venous cannula was inserted into the right atrium and connected to a bag filled with 1 L of lactated Ringer's solution. Blood and lactated Ringer's solution were equilibrated by infusing and draining the bag fluid. Emax and end-diastolic pressure-volume relation (EDPVR) were measured by rapid fluid infusion. Each Emax value without cardiac net (control) was set at 100% and compared with Emax data with cardiac net. Emax tended to increase with decreasing cardiac mesh size. In both LV and RV, statistical significance was reached at 85% of the cardiac net size. b. Relative change in diastolic stiffness constant (k) of EDPVR. Each EDPVR data point was fitted to the curve with the equation: EDP = a(ekEDV-1). Each diastolic constant k value without cardiac net (control) was set to 100% and compared to the k value with cardiac net. Diastolic constant k value tended to increase with decreasing cardiac net size. RV k-value reached statistical significance at 90% size, while LV k-value reached statistical significance at 85% size. The increase of k value in RV was greater than that in LV at 85% cardiac net size.

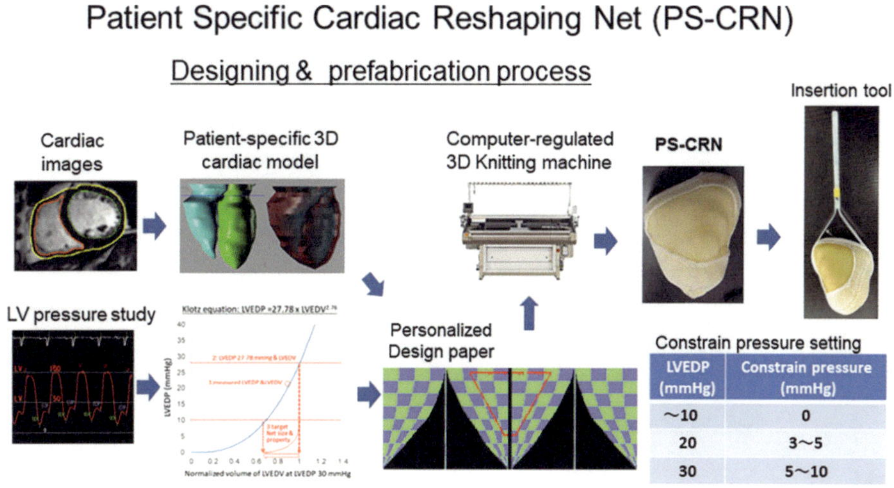

Figure 4.
Design and prefabrication process of patient- specific cardiac reshaping net (PS-CRN). (1) cardiac imaging (MRI T2 whole heart or contrast CT). (2) cardiac catheterization: Measurement of LVEDP. (3) 3D modeling of LV & RV cavity, whole ventricle surface from cardiac images (converted to STL data). (4) create design paper for computer-controlled knitting machine from 3D heart. Model (custom software: Set contact pressure 5 to 10 mmHg between LV surface and heart mesh at LVEDP 30 mmHg). (5) prefabrication of PS-CRN by computerized knitting machine.

pressure-volume ratio (LVEDPVR) in individual cases. We use the LVEDPVR estimation formula reported by Klotz et al. [12]. The concept is based on studies showing that the LVEDPVR of the human heart is almost identical when LVEDV at LVEDP 30 mmHg is normalized to 1 (normalized volume), regardless of whether the heart is normal or diseased (DCM, ICM, and HCM).

$$\begin{aligned}&\text{LVEDPVR is expressed as LVEDP} = \alpha \text{x EDV}^{\beta}\\&(\alpha = 27.78\ \text{mmHg}, \beta = 2.76\ (\text{unitless})),\\&\text{LVEDV is normalized to 1 at LVEDP 30 mmHg.}\end{aligned} \tag{1}$$

In other words, if LVEDV is set to 100% at LVEDP 30 mmHg (more precisely, at 27.78 mmHg), then LVEDP 10 mmHg is approximately 70%, 20 mmHg is approximately 80%, and 25 mmHg is 95% of the size of LVEDV at LVEDP 30 mmHg. With respect to LVEDV, the LVEDP/LVEDV ratio increases sharply as LVEDP approaches 30 mmHg. Similarly, because the PS-CRN is a knitted product, the pressure remains low just above near-unloaded sizes, but when the mesh is fully stretched, the pressure increases rapidly relative to the change in volume. The PS-CRN can be designed to prevent the heart from expanding beyond the LVEDV at LVEDP 30 mmHg by designing the mesh to be nearly fully stretched at the LVEDV size at LVEDP 30 mmHg.

Using a computer-controlled knitting machine that can produce 3D-shaped knitted products without sewing (Shima-Seiki Co. Ltd.), PS-CRN is designed and manufactured in advance for each heart failure patient according to the above concept. It is possible to safely exert sufficient pressure (>5 mmHg) on the left ventricle to improve cardiac function while avoiding right ventricular dilatation failure by making a hole in the right ventricular part.

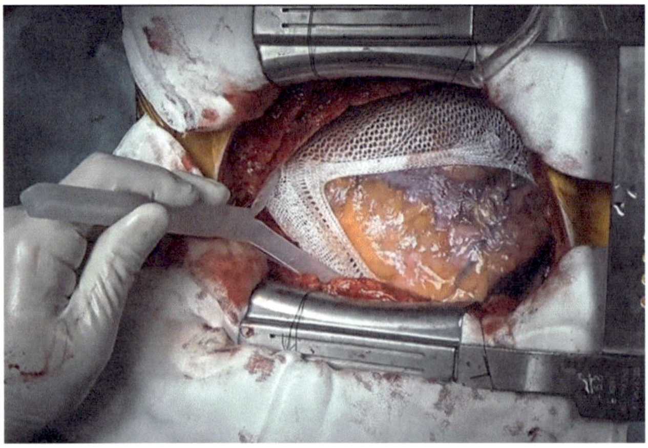

Figure 5.
Operative image of PS-CRN implantation with insertion tool. Insertion of the PS-CRN took approximately 1 minute.

	Case 1	Case 2	Case 3
gender	Male	Male	Male
Age	65	69	70
NYHA	III	III	III
INTERMACS	7	6	5
ICD/CRT-D	CRT-D	CRT-D	—
BNP (pg/ml)	111.5	111.1	1065.9
LVEDD(mm)	73.3	70.8	70.1
LVEF(%)	24.5	26.9	29.1

Table 2.
Patient demographics.

3. Implant procedure (**Figure 5**)

i. Median sternotomy or left anterior mini-thoracotomy.

ii. Insert the PS-CRN without lifting the heart using the insertion tool.

The device can be inserted through either a median sternotomy (**Figure 5**) or a left anterior thoracotomy (minimally invasive approach (MICS). Since the PS-CRN is designed and prefabricated prior to surgery, no intraoperative adjustments are required.

3. Results of first-in-human study

The first-in-human study was completed in three patients with DCM (**Table 2**) (https://jrct.niph.go.jp/en-latest-detail/jRCTs042180025). All patients are over 65 years of age, NYHA-III. UCG data showed LVDD>70 mm, LVEF<30%, and moderate mitral regurgitation. Implantation of the PS-CRN reduces left ventricular volume and mitral regurgitation to trace or mild degree during surgery. Peak oxygen consumption at

24 weeks after surgery increased by 2.8 ml/kg/min (average of 3 cases). Pulmonary wedge pressure decreased drastically (20.7 → 10.3 mmHg for average in three cases). Patients maintained a better quality of life than before surgery (preparation for submission).

We proceeded to the investigator-initiated feasibility clinical trial from June 2022 (https://jrct.niph.go.jp/en-latest-detail/jRCT2042210157). The first case had severe mitral regurgitation and pulmonary hypertension above 70 mmHg in systole at the time of surgery. Immediately after implantation, mitral regurgitation was reduced to mild, and pulmonary artery pressure dropped below 30 mmHg in systole.

4. Discussion

4.1 Current status of the patient-specific cardiac reshaping net and future direction

PS-CRN is the device that compresses the primary LV surface, the annulus of the mitral, and tricuspid valves. The amount of compression is designed by the patient's LV end-diastolic pressure-volume relationship. These two key features allow the PS-CRN to apply sufficient constraining pressure on the LV surface without compromising RV diastolic function. This direct mechanical action immediately reduces LV diastolic volume (LV reverse remodeling) and the mitral and tricuspid annulus, ultimately reducing functional mitral and tricuspid regurgitation. A first-in-human study supported these hypotheses.

With the use of the insertion tool, device implantation does not require lifting of the heart, which can cause hypotension or ventricular arrhythmias. None of the four patients in the first-in-human study required IABP or cardiopulmonary support. Insertion time in the last case was only 1 minute. The minimally invasive nature of PS-CRN implantation ensures rapid recovery from surgery.

Another advantage of this device is the ease of postoperative care. No anticoagulation or immunosuppressive medications are required, as is the case with LVADs or heart transplantation.

4.2 Limitations

The lack of randomization and the small number of patients with its possibility of bias are clear limitations in drawing definitive conclusions from our first-in-human study and need to be addressed in further studies. Another limitation is the lack of long-term results.

Future randomized trials will determine whether the observed beneficial effect is significant and sustained in patients who are maintained on evidence-based heart failure therapies over the long term.

For this reason, we believe that this device should be used preferentially in older patients until long-term results demonstrate sustained beneficial effects, such as quality of life and survival. The younger patients, who are eligible for heart transplantation, should be informed that the use of PS-CRN may increase the risk of heart transplantation. Although successful heart transplantation after CorCap implantation has been reported, the procedure required longer time for dissection of the dense adhesion of CorCap and epicardium and pericardium [13, 14].

5. Conclusion

The Patient-specific cardiac reshaping net (PS-CRN) is a pathophysiological treatment for dilated cardiomyopathy, and its reverse remodeling effect was demonstrated intraoperatively because it is designed and fabricated for each heart failure patient. The procedure was safe and fast with no device-related adverse events. The first case was followed for up to 4 years postoperatively. Initial results were promising.

6. Research funding

The first-in-human study (https://jrct.niph.go.jp/en-latest-detail/jRCTs042180025) was funded by the Terumo Foundation for Life Science and Arts.

The investigator-initiated feasibility study is funded by the Japan Agency for Medical Research and Development, Translational Research (https://jrct.niph.go.jp/en-latest-detail/jRCT2042210157).

Conflict of interest

The authors, Toshiaki Akita and Toshiya Sasaki, are co-founders, shock holders, and current board members of iCorNet Laboratory (Nagoya, Japan), the company that developed the device.

Author details

Toshiaki Akita[1,2]*, Sho Akita[1], Hideki Ito[1], Masato Mutsuga[1] and Toshiya Sasaki[2]

1 Department of Cardiac Surgery, Nagoya University Hospital, Japan

2 iCorNet Laboratory Co. Ltd., Japan

*Address all correspondence to: takita@med.nagoya-u.ac.jp

References

[1] Cohn JN, Ferrari R, Sharpe N. Cardiac remodeling–Concepts and clinical implications: A consensus paper from an international forum on cardiac remodeling. Behalf of an International Forum on Cardiac Remodeling. Journal of the American College of Cardiology. 2000;**35**(3):569-582

[2] Starling RC, Jessup M. Worldwide clinical experience with the CorCap cardiac support device. Journal of Cardiac Failure. 2004;**10**(Suppl. 6):S225-S233

[3] Mann DL et al. Clinical evaluation of the CorCap cardiac support device in patients with dilated cardiomyopathy. The Annals of Thoracic Surgery. 2007;**84**(4):1226-1235

[4] Mann DL et al. Rationale, design, and methods for a pivotal randomized clinical trial for the assessment of a cardiac support device in patients with New York health association class III-IV heart failure. Journal of Cardiac Failure. 2004;**10**(3):185-192

[5] Acker MA et al. Mitral valve surgery in heart failure: Insights from the Acorn clinical trial. The Journal of Thoracic and Cardiovascular Surgery. 2006;**132**(3):568-577

[6] Mann DL et al. Beneficial effects of the CorCap cardiac support device: Five-year results from the Acorn trial. The Journal of Thoracic and Cardiovascular Surgery. 2012;**143**(5):1036-1042

[7] Acker MA et al. Mitral valve repair in heart failure: Five-year follow-up from the mitral valve replacement stratum of the Acorn randomized trial. The Journal of Thoracic and Cardiovascular Surgery. 2011;**142**(3):569-574

[8] Mokashi SA et al. Restraint to the left ventricle alone is superior to standard restraint. The Journal of Thoracic and Cardiovascular Surgery. 2013;**146**(1):192-197

[9] Lee LS et al. Postoperative recurrence of mitral regurgitation after annuloplasty for functional mitral regurgitation. The Annals of Thoracic Surgery. 2012;**94**(4):1211-6; discussion 1216-7

[10] Okada M. Effect of cardiac support device size on right and left ventricular function in a porcine dilated heart failure model. J Kanazawa Medical University. 2015;**40**:1-10

[11] Akita T, Yamabe M, Mashiahiro S. Heart Correction Net, in US patent Office, Kanazawa Institute of Technology. Kanazawa Medical University; editor. iCorNet Laboratory: USA. 2015/0018607 A1

[12] Klotz S, Dickstein ML, Burkhoff D. A computational method of prediction of the end-diastolic pressure-volume relationship by single beat. Nature Protocols. 2007;**2**(9):2152-2158

[13] Schroder JN et al. Cardiac transplantation following ACORN CorCap device implantation. European Journal of Cardio-Thoracic Surgery. 2006;**29**(5):848-850

[14] Kawabori M et al. Successful LVAD implantation and heart transplantation after ACORN Corcap placement. Journal of Cardiac Surgery. 2019;**34**(7):624-625

Section 2

Mechanical Circulatory Support

Chapter 3

Extracorporeal Membrane Oxygenation (ECMO) Use in Heart Transplantation

Chidiebere Peter Echieh and Robert Hooker

Abstract

Extracorporeal membrane oxygenation (ECMO) use in patients both pre and post heart transplantation has become a life-saving tool in the armamentarium for physicians. Early developments in perfusion were hindered by the challenges of coagulation. Technological advances leading to contemporary management of ECMO began with the oxygenation of blood circulating through an artificial cistern. VA ECMO provides mechanical circulatory support (MCS) to patients not responding to medical treatment with primary cardiac dysfunction or combined respiratory and cardiac dysfunction failure. Management of the patient on ECMO is complex and involves multidisciplinary daily input from cardiology, cardiac surgery, and intensivist with ECMO specialization. Indications for ECMO use in heart transplantation include bridge to decision, bridge to transplant, rescue from PGD, and management of vasoplegia. The use of ECMO pre transplant has increased in the United States since the heart allocation changes implemented in 2018. Outcomes utilizing ECMO in pre and post heart transplant patients appear to be improving worldwide.

Keywords: ECMO, heart transplantation, shock, mechanical circulatory support, advanced heart failure

1. Introduction

Extracorporeal Membrane Oxygenation (ECMO) has become a vital life-saving technology in the management of advanced heart failure and heart transplant patients. Failure of optimal medical therapy in heart failure shifts the treatment options from neurohormonal modulation to surgery and palliative options. Historically, ECMO was for brief support for periods of 5–10 days however prolonged runs have been reported [1]. Contemporary use in heart failure may be classified as bridge to transplant, bridge to recovery, destination, or bridge to decision.

ECMO is employed pretransplant to provide support to patients with end-stage cardiac failure when conventional optimal medical therapy is insufficient. ECMO can be used in pure cardiac dysfunction with left, right, and biventricular failure, and unlike other mechanical options, in patients with concomitant pulmonary insufficiency due to pulmonary edema ECMO provides respiratory support. Veno-arterial extra corporeal membrane oxygenation (VA ECMO) may be utilized in neonatal, pediatric, and adult populations, making it a viable support modality for various patient populations. In the postoperative heart transplant patient, primary graft dysfunction is the most common indication for mechanical circulatory support using VA ECMO.

2. History of ECMO

Pioneering animal research on extracorporeal oxygenation began in the seventeenth century. Early experiments that included perfusion were initially limited by coagulation/thrombosis and only became possible with the development of anticoagulants. Direct contact oxygenation became available in the nineteenth century with agitated oxygenators and motorized oxygenators. Bubble-type and surface-type oxygenators were described by Hooker in the early twentieth century [2]. Following the discovery of anticoagulation, stationary screen oxygenators were developed, and subsequently modified pump oxygenators became commercially available. Rotating disc film oxygenators, which were initially developed for animal use and then adapted to human use was made possible in the mid-twentieth century. With the development of the DeWall bubble oxygenator, concerns about optimum bubble size arose. Small bubble sizes achieved a higher surface area for direct contact with blood and allowed better oxygenation; however, they had a longer transit time through the oxygenating column predisposing patients to air embolism. The best compromise was achieved with bubble sizes between 2 and 7 mm in diameter, a mixture of large- and small-sized bubbles and optimizing the rate of fresh gas flow. The use of these bubble oxygenators resulted in blood shearing with resultant hemolysis, activation of the inflammatory response, platelet activation, and increased thrombogenicity.

Technological advances that ushered in the era of contemporary ECMO began with the oxygenation of blood as it flowed through an artificial cistern. Kolf and Berk observed that the gas contents of blood approximated those of aerated dialysate across a cellophane tube [3]. This led to research on biomaterials with the hope of identifying materials with optimum gas exchange and mechanical properties. Initial materials that were tested include ethylcellulose and polyethylene, but these materials were limited by mechanical strength and presence of pinholes. The development of the membrane exchange system, the membrane lung, was made possible using polysiloxane or silicon polymers.

The development of hydrophobic, microporous membranes with pore sizes less than 1 micron, allowed direct contact of blood and air while plasmatic leak across the micropores limited by surface tension forces. These membranes allowed high-performance membrane oxygenators capable of being used for long ECMO runs.

Gibbon reported the first successful use of a mechanical extracorporeal lung and heart bypass during cardiac surgery in 1954 [4], and Hill et al. reported the first use of prolonged extracorporeal bypass in the context of post-traumatic respiratory failure in 1972 [5]. Extracorporeal support lasted for 75 hours in this case. In 1975, Bartlett went on to describe the first successful ECMO in a neonatal patient [6]. Following a premature termination of a multicenter trial of ECMO for ARDS, the development of ECMO was stalled for 20 years [7]. Thereafter, significant progress has been made in the circuit, management, indications and outcomes [8].

3. General concepts of ECMO

VA ECMO is a temporary modality of mechanical circulatory support (MCS) that can be used to support patients with pure cardiac dysfunction (RV, LV and

Biventricular) and/or combined respiratory and cardiac dysfunction failure who are refractory to optimal medical treatment. In these scenarios, ECMO is performed via a veno-arterial route. The venous drainage is from the right atrium which is usually accessed percutaneously through the femoral vein, however, the subclavian, jugular veins or a surgical central venous system may be used. Arterial cannulation can be either central/aortic or peripheral using the femoral, axillary, or subclavian artery. A recent systematic review and meta-analysis comparing central versus peripheral canulation for ECMO reports that central canulation is associated with greater hospital mortality, reoperation, and transfusion [9]. The peripheral arterial cannula range in size from 15 to 19 Fr. Central arterial cannulas are larger: up to 22 Fr. Adult-size venous cannulas used for drainage are often reinforced to avoid kinking, about 50 to 70 cm in length with a diameter of 19 to 25 FR. The presence of multiple side cannula holes along the end of the cannula facilitates drainage [10]. In pediatric patients, the sizes of the cannula are matched with the body surface area. This matching is critical to optimal delivery of support because the resistance to blood flow in the extracorporeal circuit is inversely proportional to the diameter of the return cannula [11]. Hence, optimal flows are facilitated by larger bore cannulas [12]. The ECMO circuit consists of a centrifugal pump; the oxygenator; the heat exchanger; the tubing of the circuit; the control console; the gas supply and blender; sensors and monitors; safety systems; and the power supply.

4. ECMO cannulation and management

The procedure for the institution and management of VA-ECMO support for bridge to transplant is a sterile surgical procedure and requires intravascular access with drainage and inflow cannula. This intravascular access may be achieved via the Seldinger technique or via a cut down to the target vessels. Before the commencement of ECMO, ACT should be confirmed to be greater than 200 seconds. The oxygen line is connected to the oxygenator and the gas flow set at about 5–6 L/min. The sterile loop is handed to the cannulating physician; this is cut between clamps, and the connections of the tubing to the canulae are made to the exclusion of air. Flows are adjusted to maintain mean arterial pressure and adequate arterial oxygenation. Baseline ventilator requirements and anticoagulation sampling times are determined. The lines are secured as required using anchoring sutures and Opsite® (Smith and Nephew). Typical ventilatory setting may include FiO_2 less than 70%, positive inspiratory pressure less than 35cmH_2O, PEEP of <10, and respiratory rate < 10. Typical flow rates for a VA-ECMO would be in the range of 2.1 to 2.4 L/min/M^2. Prolonged flow rates less than 2 liters should be avoided as this predisposes to thrombosis. Pre-membrane pressures should be kept below 300 mmHg to avoid catastrophic line accidents. Target transmembrane gradient should be less than 50 mmHg. The circuit should be changed if transmembrane gradient is above 150 mmHg as this may be due to clot formation and/or fibrin accumulation in the oxygenator. The ECMO pumps are almost exclusively centrifugal pumps and consist of a rotor that drives blood on rotation. Contemporary oxygenators are commonly Quadrox® (Getinge) or Nautilus® (Medtronic) oxygenators. The Quadrox® (Getinge) oxygenator uses hollow fiber membranes for gas exchange and have a compact design that integrates the heat exchanger with the oxygenator. The Nautilus® (Medtronic) oxygenator uses hollow fiber or flat sheet membranes for gas exchange and has a modular design with separate heat exchanger and oxygenator. Understanding these designs will assist healthcare providers customize the set up to individual patient needs.

Signs of limb mal perfusion as well as differential perfusion as seen in Harlequin syndrome should be monitored for and documented. Harlequin syndrome results from blood flow through the heart that is not oxygenated, because of lung pathology, being ejected to upper body. The oxygenated blood which is delivered back to body through a groin cannula meets the unoxygenated blood near the distal arch. Coronary and brain perfusion may be compromised. It is imperative to monitor PaO2/ SaO2 in right upper extremity. For ECMO-Impella combination therapy, the cannulation strategy involves a standard femoral or central cannulation for ECMO while the Impella device may be deployed through the femoral or subclavian artery. Typically, the Impella is deployed on the contralateral side of the ECMO cannulation site.

Other parameters monitored include temperature with a goal of maintenance of normothermia using the heater - cooler. ACT/ aPTT guided titration of heparin dosing should be done 6-hourly for the first 24 hours. Following the exclusion of reactionary hemorrhage, ACT may be lowered from commencement levels of above 200 to about 150 if platelet counts are stable. Measurement every six hours aPTT with a target of 40 to 80 seconds should be used to monitor patient subsequently. Direct thrombin inhibitors such as Bivalirudin may be used in cases of heparin resistance requiring frequent antithrombin III replacement or heparin-induced thrombocytopenia. Serum lactate, renal function hepatic function and daily wake up assessment should be monitored according to institutional protocols.

While VA ECMO improves systemic flow and unloads the right ventricle it does increase LV afterload. The LV is subjected to significant increases in afterload from blood being pumped backwards toward the aortic valve. This may lead to a loss of pulsatility, aortic valve closure, and if aortic insufficiency is present LV distension and transmural ischemia and increasing LVEDP and eventually pulmonary edema. Decreased aortic valve opening, LV distention and stasis can cause LV cavity thrombosis and subsequent strokes and peripheral artery embolic events. Careful monitoring for left-sided distension is required using chest x-rays, attention to ventilator plateau pressures and oxygenation needs, as well as assessment of pulmonary artery pressures using a pulmonary catheter, and frequent echocardiographic assessment. Early treatment with inotropes may be sufficient, however with continued LV distension, further interventions may be necessary. Intra-aortic balloon counter pulsation reduces after load and may be easily inserted in ICU. The placement of a LV axial flow pump, (Impella ® (Abiomed)) is an excellent way to achieve decompression. This may be done in the Cath lab or the OR under fluoroscopic guidance. If a patient has prosthetic aortic valve, percutaneous pulmonary artery vents can be placed or surgical vents which are less desirable because of the incision with bleeding consequences. Prevention, rather than treatment, of these complications should be the rule and routine use of LV unloading early during an ECMO run with an LV axial flow pump is strongly encouraged.

5. ECMO use in heart transplantation

Extracorporeal Membrane Oxygenation (ECMO) can play a crucial role in heart transplantation by providing temporary circulatory and, if necessary, respiratory support to patients pre- and/ or post transplantation.

5.1 Bridge to decision

In patients presenting in cardiogenic shock, emergency ECMO may be used to resuscitate and support the cardiovascular system while the patient is evaluated for multiple decision pathways including transplant, durable MCS, shifted palliative care or achieve recovery from shock and are weaned off VA ECMO. The availability and speed of deployment of VA ECMO makes it the circulatory support device of choice in emergent potentially terminal cardiac events such as refractory ventricular fibrillation arrests, refractory cardiogenic shock, and pulseless electrical activity. Use of ECMO prior to determination of subsequent treatment options, which may include transplantation, is referred to as bridge to decision. It is notable that, in a significant proportion of patients, sufficient recovery occurs to allow weaning from the ECMO support [13].

5.2 Bridge to transplant (BTT)

ECMO use as a bridge to transplantation is most commonly used for patients already on the wait list, as opposed to those placed on the wait list while already on ECMO [14–17]. By providing mechanical support of the heart, ECMO allows patients to stabilize and recover from cardiogenic shock refractory to maximal medical management, while waiting for a suitable donor organ to become available. This not only increases their chances of successful transplantation but also reduces the risk of further complications and end organ deterioration. Notably, ECMO improves renal and hepatic perfusion, with the goal of normalization of function prior to transplant [18]. This support not only helps stabilize the patient's condition but elevates their status on the transplant waiting list.

5.3 Rescue from primary graft dysfunction (PGD)

Primary graft dysfunction is identified when the transplanted allograft fails to function adequately in the early postoperative period [19]. PGD may be at least partially attributable to ischemia-reperfusion injury of the graft, immunological response and from a combination of other host and donor factors. It is recognized as a low cardiac output state, with potentially pulmonary edema and/ or arrhythmias. The right ventricle, left ventricle, or biventricular involvement can occur. Initial management involves expansion of intravascular volume and use of inotropes; however these may not suffice and, unhindered, may lead to multiple organ dysfunction. Rescue treatment by use of VA ECMO support maintains perfusion and oxygenation while the graft recovery occurs. Peripheral cannulation support in PGD was associated with better survival then central [20].

5.4 Management of Persistent Vasoplegia

Vasoplegia occurs when systemic vasodilation with consequent hypotension complicates the hemodynamics in the post CPB/post-transplant period. It is at least partially attributable to unregulated release of nitric oxide from reperfusion injury. This syndrome leads to severe hypotension refractory to high doses of vasopressors, despite normal appearing cardiac function. The hypotension and high dose vasopressors have deleterious effect on end organ perfusion. Medical management includes fluid therapy, Vitamin B12, vasopressors including Angiotensin II, and intravenous methylene blue. VA ECMO support should be instituted in persistent vasoplegia as a rescue therapy when medical management fails to restore adequate perfusion to prevent end organ failure.

6. ECMO as a bridge to transplant

Worldwide, changes to heart allocation guidelines prioritize patients on mechanical circulatory support, including ECMO. This new allocation system became effective in the United States in 2018, in the United Kingdom in 2016, and in France in 2004. Since then, there has been an increasing use of VA-ECMO as a bridge to heart transplant worldwide. Across the United States, the use of VA-ECMO as a direct bridge to heart transplant increased from 1.1% in 2012 to 5.2 in 2022 [21, 22]. Advanced heart failure has remained the most common indication in patients who receive VA-ECMO as a bridge to transplant. Unfortunately, the term “advanced heart failure” is not clearly defined. Patients with advanced heart failure can be identified by signs of circulatory failure with attendant renal and hepatic dysfunction, frequent malignant arrhythmias, and the need for continuous intravenous inotropes. Options for mechanical circulatory support include the Intra-Aortic Balloon Pump (IABP), various ventricular assist devices (VAD), VA ECMO and Impella ® (Abiomed). The choice of device for support is based on patient factors as well as available technology and expertise, residual left ventricular function, right ventricular function, pulmonary artery pressures, status of the aortic valve and need to unload the left ventricle. Bridging to transplant with ECMO has been considered controversial and not preferred because, compared to VAD, it requires immobilization, anticoagulation, and ICU care. Also, there is a high rate of waitlist mortality in patients bridged to transplant with ECMO. This practice is associated with a survival to hospital discharge rate of less than 50% [23].

The versatility and efficacy in delivering biventricular as well as pulmonary support has continued to earn its place as an option for MCS delivery. In addition, the speed of deployment makes it suitable for emergency situations, such as critical sudden circulatory collapse. In an analysis of the post 2018 allocation change in the United States, 3.6% of transplants were on ECMO (bridge to decision) at the time of listing and 5.2% of transplants in the same period were on ECMO at transplantation (bridge to transplant) [21]. The success of ECMO bridging to heart transplant or VAD is estimated to be between 44 and 79% with the most prevalent complications estimated to include bleeding (46%), arrhythmia (26%), device thrombus (24%), and device malfunction (23%) [24–26].

Several centers have reported bridging to transplant with ECMO as a risk factor for worse post-transplant survival. An analysis of the UNOS database by Moonsamy et al. showed that bridging with ECMO was a significant predictor of post-transplant mortality with lower 1 year survival rate of transplants bridged on ECMO (68 vs. 90%) [27]. In a similar analysis by Fukuhara et al. ECMO as direct bridge to transplant demonstrated lower posttransplant survival compared with continuous flow LVAD with survival rates of 73.1 versus 93.1% at 90 days, and 67.4 versus 82.4% at 3 years respectively [16]. These results reflect the acuity of patients on ECMO and the attendant issues with coagulation, end-organ perfusion, deconditioning, debility and inflammatory response associated with VA ECMO support.

Aimed at reducing the afterload, ECMO support may be combined with Impella support in a combined mechanical circulatory support known as ECMO-Impella combination therapy or ECPELLA, this has been used in cases of cardiogenic shock and was reported to be associated with activation of cardioprotective signaling [28]. The addition of Impella to ECMO support is based on the finding that, in contrast to ECMO, Impella reduces infarct size [29]. Hence the opinion that left ventricular unloading may mitigate myocardial injury in patients on ECMO. Delivery of hemodynamic support is done by titrating flow rates of the devices while avoiding complications. Weaning protocols for ECPELLA are individualized according to patients' clinical context. Generally, in patients who are bridged to heart transplant and in whom ECMO component of combined therapy was used to provide respiratory support, weaning the ECMO first may be favored as the lung recovers. While in patients who bridged for heart and lung transplant due to pulmonary failure and failure of both ventricles, weaning the Impella first would be the goal.

In a retrospective review of ECPELLA use in cardiogenic shock, Patel et al. reported that 30-day mortality was significantly lower in the ECPELLA cohort compared with the VA-ECMO cohort, this difference remained significant after adjusting for STEMI and PCI [30]. Also, one-year all-cause mortality was significantly lower in the ECPELLA group. The use of ECPELLA was associated with higher rates of hemolysis and need for hemofiltration [31].

Reviews of the practice of VA ECMO bridge to heart transplant in the United States since the 2018 change in UNOS allocation policy shows that there has been an increase in the use of temporary MCS, including ECMO, following the policy change [21, 32]. This increase in the use of temporary MCS was noted to have occurred in transplant centers but not in other critical care units, despite similar patient characteristics during two time periods. The allocation system may have driven a change in practitioners' behavior, not the patients [33]. Considering outcomes, Cogswell et al., Trivedi et al., as well as Kilic et al. reported a decrease in unadjusted post-transplant survival following the policy change [34–36]. Goff et al. reported no difference in unadjusted post-transplant survival following the policy change [37]. In contrast, patients supported on ECMO following the most recent allocation policy change were more likely to receive heart transplants, and less likely to die on the waitlist or be removed from the waitlist; they also had a lower average waitlist time [38].

These varying results may be attributable to informative censoring. More transplant candidates are waitlisted on ECMO since the most recent allocation policy change, however the demographics of patients waitlisted on ECMO did not change with the new policy. Comparatively, a greater percentage of ECMO bridges are undergoing transplant in the new era compared to the old allocation policy (78.6 vs. 37.6%). Following transplantation, 90-day survival in ECMO bridged patients were comparable in the two eras with a nonsignificant decrease in 1 year survival in the new era [14].

Kim et al. noted that there was improved waitlist and post-transplant outcomes in patients bridged with ECMO following the most recent change in heart allocation policy [39]. In their report, bridging with ECMO was strongly associated with worse 1-year mortality prior to the policy change, while ECMO patients transplanted after the policy change have similar post-transplant outcomes as non-ECMO patients. They concluded that their findings suggest that ECMO may be most effective as a bridging modality when patients are transplanted promptly following initial listing. There is also a possibility that nonrestrictive patient selection for ECMO bridging may be a possible alternative explanation. Despite these issues, when deaths within first 30 days of transplant were excluded, the use of ECMO was not associated with increased mortality [40, 41].

Predictors of failure of the ECMO bridge to transplant have been reported to include left ventricular EF, older age, ischemic heart disease, pre-ECMO cardiopulmonary resuscitation, and high Sequential Organ Failure Assessment (SOFA) scores [42, 43]. Other factors associated with failure include the presence of female sex, dilated cardiomyopathy, decompensated heart failure, the occurrence of complications such as stroke, and the need for dialysis [24]. There is little hope that a complete consensus will soon be reached on the age limit for successful bridging. Smedira et al. recommend 60 years with decompensated heart failure, while Chung et al. [43, 44] recommend 50 years with a SOFA score of 10. Analyses of the organ procurement and transplant network data on ECMO bridges in the pediatric population in the US showed that 45% of the cohort bridged on ECMO survived to transplantation, 10% of the cohort recovered enough to be removed from the waitlist, 11% were removed from waitlist due to clinical deterioration and 28% died while on the waiting list [24].

In an analysis of use of ECMO bridge to transplant by Dong et al., median bridging time in the BTT group was 13 days (interquartile range [IQR], 7–19 days) [45]. Generally, ECMO support longer than 14 days is a risk factor for posttransplant mortality [24, 46]. It is important to note that while ECMO is reliable for temporary bridge to transplantation, it is not an option for long-term mechanical circulatory support to bridge transplant candidates. When full flow on ECMO for more than a few days is required to achieve adequate organ perfusion, escalation of ECMO to LVAD provides a safe and durable support that provides cardiac unloading, high flow, and physiological circulatory patterns [47].

Outside the United States, experience with the use of ECMO as bridge for heart transplantation showed that, comparatively, temporary left ventricular assist devices were associated with a lower risk of death in the first year of the bridge when compared with VA-ECMO [25]. The higher mortality noted in patients who were bridged with VA-ECMO could be attributable to the higher prevalence of critically ill patients and more adverse events in the ECMO group [35].

In the United Kingdom, VA-ECMO bridge-to-transplant is uncommon, while temporary LVAD such as Impella ® (Abiomed), make up the vast majority of bridged patients. In a review following the change in allocation system, only a handful of patients were bridged using VA-ECMO [48].

Analysis of the French national registry shows ECMO bridged patients to have higher priority and shows that patients bridged with ECMO have higher incidence of being dependent on intravenous inotropes, mechanical ventilation, and dialysis. Despite these features suggesting higher acuity among heart transplant patients bridged on ECMO, French patients bridged on VA-ECMO had a comparably good outcome with equivalent mortality in single center analyses [49] and even lower risk of mortality in national database analysis [50]. Notably, the duration of extracorporeal life support was short with a mean duration of 6.3 ± 4.6 days [15].

7. Indications for ECMO bridge to transplant

Indications for ECMO bridge to transplant are not different from published indications for mechanical circulatory support, namely, advanced heart failure with progression of failure despite optimal medical therapy. The American Heart Association admits that there is no consensus on the definition of advanced heart failure [51]. This leaves practitioners to identify patients with advanced heart failure by the presence of subjective features such as the requirement for critical care, continuous ionotropic requirements, and consideration for heart transplantation, MCS, or hospice. Objective assessments, where used, include measures of functional limitation such as peak Vo2 of ≤14 (or < 50% of expected) mL/kg/min and a 6-minute walk of less than 300 meters. In practice, it is often not feasible to determine these objective assessments at the time the decision to institute ECMO support is made. The ideal scenario would be for the shock team to make the decision even in emergent cases, based on the clinical state of the patient.

After failure of medical therapy, options for effective therapy are limited to mechanical circulatory support, heart transplant and palliative care. Due to the scarcity of donor organs, temporary or durable mechanical circulatory support becomes the default option in the absence of donor hearts. When patients require both cardiac and pulmonary support, VA ECMO is the only option.

8. Post-operative ECMO use in heart transplantation

Indications for the use of ECMO mechanical circulatory support following a heart transplant include the occurrence of hyperacute graft rejection, post-operative bleeding, severe vasoplegia, and primary graft dysfunction.

Hyperacute rejection occurs within minutes to hours following a heart transplant, results from an antibody-mediated rejection (AMR) in response to HLA donor specific antibodies, and results in rapid damage to the graft with deposition of C4d complement. The diagnosis of antibody mediated rejection was previously, made in cases of graft dysfunction in the absence of cellular rejection. Recently, the requirement of histological evidence of antibody mediated injury was included [52, 53]. This inclusion helps to differentiate hyperacute rejection from non-immunological causes (NIC) of graft dysfunction. Notably, transplant guidelines recognize that AMR may occur when neither donor specific antibodies nor C4d deposition is present. Both AMR and NIC may present with severe pulmonary edema, profound coagulopathy, and biventricular failure. With current practice of HLA matching, hyper-acute rejection due to AMR has become rare [54, 55]. There are still instances of hyperacute graft dysfunction in orthotopic heart transplantation in the presence of non-HLA antibodies. These have been attributed to anti-angiotensin type I receptor antibodies [56].

The entities of vasoplegia and PGD after orthotopic heart transplantation have significant overlap with both conditions having a common factor of severely reduced afterload. It is possible that either entity may be complicated by the other for example, the increased capacity of the vascular system resulting from loss of vascular tone and attendant vasodilation as seen in vasoplegia may, in the presence of a denervated heart and loss of cardioaccelerator response, lead to ineffective cardiac output and resulting fall in afterload. The resulting cardiovascular collapse leads to failure of coronary perfusion and other end-organs. PGD which may result from myocardial stunning, leading to inadequate cardiac output which is beyond the capacity of the initial vasoconstrictive response to maintain cardiac afterload. The report of increase in PGD with longer ischemic time supports the second theory [57, 58]. A third possibility is autonomic dyssynergia between the denervated cardioaccelerator beta 1 supply to the heart and the vasoconstrictive alpha supply to the vascular system.

Regardless of the pathogenesis, the use of a VA-ECMO in patients with severe primary graft dysfunction and/or vasoplegia following heart transplantation is recommended in situations of escalating inotropes and poor ventricular function [59–61]. VA-ECMO empties the right heart, allows systemic circulatory support and increases afterload makes this modality an appropriate technology for the management of PGD and vasoplegia. Pressure dynamics following institution of VA ECMO may result in failure of the passive aortic valve to open due to the continuous pressurization of the aorta above the left ventricular pressure. This could result in LV stasis and thrombosis [62]. Failure of left ventricular emptying may result in distension and increased wall tension, decrease of subendocardial perfusion and perpetuate the graft failure [63]. The target should be to prevent rather than treat ECMO related complications in the post-transplant period.

9. Weaning

Following satisfactory cardiac recovery evidenced by minimal inotropic support, maintenance of pulse pressure greater than 15 mmHg, and MAP above 65 mmHg at ECMO flow rate of 2 L/min; the patient is considered for weaning from the ECMO support. Prior to this it is imperative to ensure that bleeding has resolved, any indication for delayed sternal closure should have been resolved, and central venous pressure should be within acceptable limits.

Several successful protocols have been employed for successful VA ECMO weaning. Once such protocol involves a turn down test performed under TEE guidance. The process of weaning consists of reducing the flow rate by 50% for 10 minutes; then, if the right and left ventricular EF do not deteriorate and no mitral regurgitation or distension of the left ventricle occurs, an additional 25% reduction of flow support is done for 5 minutes. If at this time, the TEE demonstrates good function, then weaning may commence. Recognizing that even minimal ECMO flows decompress, and hence may not completely test, the right heart function; the interim ELSO guideline on VA ECMO recommends Pump Controlled Retrograde Trial where the arterial flow probe is reversed, and 1 liter of flow is returned to the right heart through the venous cannula. Successful weaning is expected following a turn down test evidenced by mean arterial pressure above sixty mm Hg, left ventricular outflow track velocity time integral (VTI) above 0.12 m/s, tissue Doppler lateral mitral annulus peak systolic velocity of 6 cm/second and above, central veinous pressure of ≤10 mm Hg, and left ventricular EF ≥ 25–30% on minimal doses of one or two inotropes or pressors [64].

Another weaning protocol consists of progressively reducing the support daily and at least a daily TEE check. In this protocol, the support is initially reduced to 75% support for 24 hours, if the hemodynamics remain stable, a TEE is performed to confirm that ejection fraction remains greater than 40% with no left ventricular distension and MR. Weaning is advanced by further reduction to 50% support for 24 hours, and then 40% while ensuring stable vitals, inotropes and labs. It is acceptable to decannulate if parameters remain stable with 25% support for one hour [59].

10. Summary

In summary, ECMO is a valuable tool for mechanical circulatory support in heart transplant patients. The development of ECMO has a rich history that continues to advance the care of critically ill patients before heart transplant, and in cases with post-op catastrophic complications that were hitherto certain mortality. Advancements in anticoagulation and extracorporeal oxygenation have been fundamental to the development of this technology.

Author details

Chidiebere Peter Echieh[1] and Robert Hooker[2]*

1 Division of Cardiothoracic Surgery, Department of Surgery, University of Calabar, Nigeria

2 Surgery Corewell Health, Michigan State University College of Human Medicine, Michigan, USA

*Address all correspondence to: drbobhooker@gmail.com

References

[1] Flinspach AN, Raimann FJ, Bauer F, Zacharowski K, Ippolito A, Booke H. Therapy and outcome of prolonged Veno-venous ECMO therapy of critically ill ARDS patients. Journal of Clinical Medicine. 2023;**12**(7):2499. DOI: 10.3390/jcm12072499

[2] Lim MW. The history of extracorporeal oxygenators. Anaesthesia. 2006;**61**(10):984-995

[3] Kolff WJ, Berk HT, ter Welle M, van der LEY AJ, van Dijk EC, van Noordwijk J. The artificial kidney: A dialyser with a great area. 1944. Journal of the American Society of Nephrology. Dec 1997;**8**(12):1959-1965. DOI: 10.1681/ASN.V8121959. PMID: 9402100

[4] Hewitt RL, Creech O. History of the Pump Oxygenator. Available from: http://archsurg.jamanetwork.com/

[5] Hill DJ, O'Brien TG, Murray JJ, Dontigny L, Bramson ML, Osborn JJ, et al. Prolonged extracorporeal oxygenation for acute post traumatic respiratory failure (shock lung syndrome). The New England Journal of Medicine. 1972;**286**(12):629-672

[6] Bartlett RH. Esperanza. Presidential address. Transactions of the American Society for Artificial Internal Organs. 1985;**31**:723-726. PMID: 3915623

[7] Bartlett RH, Gazzaniga AB, Jefferies MR, Huxtable RF, Haiduc NJ, Fong SW. Extracorporeal membrane oxygenation (ECMO) cardiopulmonary support in infancy. Transactions of the American Society for Artificial Internal Organs. 1976;**22**:80-93. PMID: 951895

[8] Bartlett RH, Gazzaniga AB, Fong SW, Jefferies MR, Roohk HV, Haiduc N. Extracorporeal membrane oxygenator support for cardiopulmonary failure experience in 28 cases. The Journal of Thoracic and Cardiovascular Surgery. 1977;**73**(3):375-386

[9] Mariscalco G, Salsano A, Fiore A, Dalén M, Ruggieri VG, Saeed D, et al. Peripheral versus central extracorporeal membrane oxygenation for postcardiotomy shock: Multicenter registry, systematic review, and meta-analysis. Journal of Thoracic and Cardiovascular Surgery. 2020;**160**(5):1207-1216.e44

[10] Patroniti N, Grasselli G, Pesenti A. Extracorporeal support of gas exchange. In: Murray and Nadel's Textbook of Respiratory Medicine. Amsterdam: Elsevier; 2016. pp. 1794-1806

[11] Chaves RC d F, Rabello Filho R, Timenetsky KT, Moreira FT, Vilanova LC d S, Bravim B d A, et al. Extracorporeal membrane oxygenation: A literature review. Revista Brasileira de Terapia Intensiva. 2019;**31**(3):410-424

[12] Pavlushkov E, Berman M, Valchanov K. Cannulation techniques for extracorporeal life support. Annals of Translational Medicine. Feb 2017;**5**(4):70. DOI: 10.21037/atm.2016.11.47. PMID: 28275615; PMCID: PMC5337209

[13] Rousse N, Juthier F, Pinçon C, Hysi I, Banfi C, Robin E, et al. ECMO as a bridge to decision: Recovery, VAD, or heart transplantation? International Journal of Cardiology. 2015;**187**(1):620-627

[14] Hess NR, Hickey GW, Sultan I, Kilic A. Extracorporeal membrane oxygenation bridge to heart transplant: Trends following the allocation change. Journal of Cardiac Surgery. 2021;**36**(1):40-47

[15] Barth E, Durand M, Heylbroeck C, Rossi-Blancher M, Boignard A, Vanzetto G, et al. Extracorporeal life support as a bridge to high-urgency heart transplantation. Clinical Transplantation. 2012;**26**(3):484-488

[16] Fukuhara S, Takeda K, Kurlansky PA, Naka Y, Takayama H. Extracorporeal membrane oxygenation as a direct bridge to heart transplantation in adults. Journal of Thoracic and Cardiovascular Surgery. 2018;**155**(4):1607-1618.e6. DOI: 10.1016/j.jtcvs.2017.10.152

[17] Šipuš D, Krželj K, Đurić Ž, Gašparović H, Miličić D, Hanževački JŠ, et al. Veno-arterial extracorporeal membrane oxygenation as a bridge to heart transplant—Change of paradigm. Journal of Clinical Medicine. 30 Nov 2022;**11**:(23):7101. DOI: 10.3390/jcm11237101. PMID: 36498676; PMCID: PMC9736223

[18] Saito S, Shibasaki I, Matsuoka T, Niitsuma K, Hirota S, Kanno Y, et al. Impella support as a bridge to heart surgery in patients with cardiogenic shock. Interactive Cardiovascular and Thoracic Surgery. 9 Jul 2022;**35**(2):ivac088. DOI: 10.1093/icvts/ivac088. PMID: 35373286; PMCID: PMC9297506

[19] Listijono DR, Watson A, Pye R, Keogh AM, Kotlyar E, Spratt P, et al. Usefulness of extracorporeal membrane oxygenation for early cardiac allograft dysfunction. Journal of Heart and Lung Transplantation. 2011;**30**(7):783-789

[20] Olivella A, Almenar-Bonet L, González-Vilchez F, Díez-López C, Díaz-Molina B, Blázquez-Bermejo Z, et al. Mechanical circulatory support in severe primary graft dysfunction: Peripheral cannulation but not earlier implantation improves survival in heart transplantation. Journal of Heart and Lung Transplantation. 2023;**42**(8):1101-1111

[21] Echieh CP, Hamidi M, Rogers M, Kazui T, Hooker R. Use of mechanical circulatory support in orthotopic heart transplantation: A 10-year analysis. The Journal of Heart and Lung Transplantation. 2023;**42**(4):S23

[22] Van Diepen S, Katz JN, Albert NM, Henry TD, Jacobs AK, Kapur NK, et al. American heart association council on clinical cardiology; Council on cardiovascular and stroke nursing; council on quality of care and outcomes research; and mission: lifeline. Contemporary management of cardiogenic shock: A scientific statement from the american heart association. Circulation. 17 Oct 2017;**136**(16):e232-e268. DOI: 10.1161/CIR.0000000000000525. Epub 2017 Sep 18. PMID: 28923988

[23] Jeewa A, Manlhiot C, McCrindle BW, Van Arsdell G, Humpl T, Dipchand AI. Outcomes with ventricular assist device versus extracorporeal membrane oxygenation as a bridge to Pediatric heart transplantation. Artificial Organs. 2010;**34**(12):1087-1091

[24] Almond CS, Singh TP, Gauvreau K, Piercey GE, Fynn-Thompson F, Rycus PT, et al. Extracorporeal membrane oxygenation for bridge to heart transplantation among children in the United States: Analysis of data from the organ procurement and transplant network and extracorporeal life support organization registry. Circulation. 2011;**123**(25):2975-2984

[25] Barge-Caballero E, Almenar-Bonet L, Gonzalez-Vilchez F, Lambert-Rodríguez JL, González-Costello J, Segovia-Cubero J, et al. Clinical outcomes of temporary mechanical circulatory support as a direct bridge to heart transplantation: A nationwide Spanish registry.

European Journal of Heart Failure. 2018;**20**(1):178-186

[26] Blume ED, Naftel DC, Bastardi HJ, Duncan BW, Kirklin JK, Webber SA. Outcomes of children bridged to heart transplantation with ventricular assist devices: A multi-institutional study. Circulation. 2006;**113**(19):2313-2319

[27] Moonsamy P, Axtell AL, Ibrahim NE, Funamoto M, Tolis G, Lewis GD, et al. Survival after heart transplantation in patients bridged with mechanical circulatory support. Journal of the American College of Cardiology. 2020;**75**(23):2892-2905

[28] Ekanem E, Gattani R, Bakhshi H, Tehrani B, Batchelor W. Combined Venoarterial ECMO and Impella-CP circulatory support for cardiogenic shock due to papillary muscle rupture. JACC Case Reports. 2020;**2**(14):2169-2172

[29] Everett KD, Swain L, Reyelt L, Majumdar M, Qiao X, Bhave S, et al. Transvalvular unloading mitigates ventricular injury due to venoarterial extracorporeal membrane oxygenation in acute myocardial infarction. JACC: Basic to Translational Science. 2023;**8**(7):769-780

[30] Patel SM, Lipinski J, Al-Kindi SG, Patel T, Saric P, Li J, et al. Simultaneous venoarterial extracorporeal membrane oxygenation and percutaneous left ventricular decompression therapy with impella is associated with improved outcomes in refractory cardiogenic shock. ASAIO Journal. 2019;**65**(1):21-28

[31] Pappalardo F, Schulte C, Pieri M, Schrage B, Contri R, Soeffker G, et al. Concomitant implantation of Impella® on top of veno-arterial extracorporeal membrane oxygenation may improve survival of patients with cardiogenic shock. European Journal of Heart Failure. 2017;**19**(3):404-412

[32] Varshney AS, Hirji SA, Givertz MM. Outcomes in the 2018 UNOS donor heart allocation system : A perspective on disparate analyses. Journal of Heart and Lung Transplantation. 2020;**39**(11):1191-1194. DOI: 10.1016/j.healun.2020.08.012

[33] Varshney AS, Berg DD, Katz JN, Baird-Zars VM, Bohula EA, Carnicelli AP, et al. Use of temporary mechanical circulatory support for Management of Cardiogenic Shock before and after the united network for organ sharing donor heart allocation system changes. JAMA Cardiology. 2020;**5**(6):703-708

[34] Cogswell R, John R, Estep JD, Duval S, Tedford RJ, Pagani FD, et al. An early investigation of outcomes with the new 2018 donor heart allocation system in the United States. Journal of Heart and Lung Transplantation. 2020;**39**(1):1-4

[35] Kilic A, Hickey G, Mathier MA, Kormos RL, Sultan I, Gleason TG, et al. Outcomes of the first 1300 adult heart transplants in the United States after the allocation policy change. Circulation. 2020;**141**(20):1662-1664

[36] Trivedi JR, Slaughter MS. "Unintended" consequences of changes in heart transplant allocation policy: Impact on practice patterns. ASAIO Journal. 2020;**66**(2):125-127

[37] Goff RR, Uccellini K, Lindblad K, Hall S, Davies R, Farr M, et al. A change of heart : Preliminary results of the US 2018 adult heart allocation revision. American Journal of Transplantation. 2020;**20**(10):2781-2790. DOI: 10.1111/ajt.16010

[38] Gonzalez MH, Acharya D, Lee S, Leacche M, Boeve T, Manandhar-Shrestha N, et al. Improved survival after heart transplantation in patients bridged with extracorporeal

membrane oxygenation in the new allocation system. Journal of Heart and Lung Transplantation. 2021;**40**(2):149-157

[39] Kim ST, Xia Y, Tran Z, Hadaya J, Dobaria V, Choi CW, et al. Outcomes of extracorporeal membrane oxygenation following the 2018 adult heart allocation policy. PLoS One. 2022;**17**(5):e0268771. DOI: 10.1371/journal.pone.0268771. PMID: 35594315; PMCID: PMC9122227

[40] Marasco SF, Vale M, Pellegrino V, Preovolos A, Leet A, Kras A, et al. Extracorporeal membrane oxygenation in primary graft failure after heart transplantation. Annals of Thoracic Surgery. 2010;**90**(5):1541-1546

[41] Zalawadiya S, Fudim M, Bhat G, Cotts W, Lindenfeld JA. Extracorporeal membrane oxygenation support and post-heart transplant outcomes among United States adults. Journal of Heart and Lung Transplantation. 2017;**36**(1):77-81

[42] Cusanno A, Aissaoui N, Minville V, Porterie J, Biendel C, Volle K, et al. Predictors of weaning failure in case of VA ECMO implantation. Scientific Reports. 16 Aug 2022;**12**(1):13842. DOI: 10.1038/s41598-022-18105-y. PMID: 35974037; PMCID: PMC9381562

[43] Chung JCY, Tsai PR, Chou NK, Chi NH, Wang SS, Ko WJ. Extracorporeal membrane oxygenation bridge to adult heart transplantation. Clinical Transplantation. 2010;**24**(3):375-380

[44] Smedira NG, Moazami N, Golding CM, McCarthy PM, Apperson-Hansen C, Blackstone EH, et al. Clinical experience with 202 adults receiving extracorporeal membrane oxygenation for cardiac failure: Survival at five years. Journal of Thoracic and Cardiovascular Surgery. 2001;**122**(1):92-102

[45] Oh DK, Hong SB, Shim TS, Kim DK, Choi S, Lee GD, et al. Effects of the duration of bridge to lung transplantation with extracorporeal membrane oxygenation. PLoS One. 2021;**16**(7):e0253520

[46] Nasir BS, Klapper J, Hartwig M. Lung transplant from ECMO: Current results and predictors of post-transplant mortality. Current Transplantation Reports. 2021;**8**:140-150. DOI: 10.1007/s40472-021-00323-4

[47] Tarzia V, Bagozzi L, Ponzoni M, Bortolussi G, Folino G, Bianco R, et al. How to optimize ECLS results beyond ventricular unloading: From ECMO to CentriMag® eVAD. Journal of Clinical Medicine. 7 Aug 2022;**11**(15):4605. DOI: 10.3390/jcm11154605. PMID: 35956219; PMCID: PMC9369484

[48] Rushton S, Parameshwar J, Lim S, Dar O, Callan P, Al-Attar N, et al. The introduction of a super-urgent heart allocation scheme in the UK: A 2-year review. Journal of Heart and Lung Transplantation. 2020;**39**(10):1109-1117

[49] Coutance G, Jacob N, Demondion P, Nguyen LS, Bouglé A, Bréchot N, et al. Favorable outcomes of a direct heart transplantation strategy in selected patients on extracorporeal membrane oxygenation support. Critical Care Medicine. 2020;**48**(4):498-506

[50] Jasseron C, Lebreton G, Cantrelle C, Legeai C, Leprince P, Flecher E, et al. Impact of heart transplantation on survival in patients on venoarterial extracorporeal membrane oxygenation at listing in France. Transplantation. 2016;**100**(9):1979-1987

[51] Peura JL, Colvin-Adams M, Francis GS, Grady KL, Hoffman TM, Jessup M, et al. Recommendations for the use of mechanical circulatory

support: Device strategies and patient selection: A scientific statement from the American heart association. Circulation. 2012;**126**(22):2648-2667

[52] Levine DJ, Glanville AR, Aboyoun C, Belperio J, Benden C, Berry GJ, et al. Antibody-mediated rejection of the lung: A consensus report of the International Society for Heart and Lung Transplantation. Journal of Heart and Lung Transplantation. 2016;**35**(4):397-406

[53] Reed EF, Demetris AJ, Hammond E, Itescu S, Kobashigawa JA, Reinsmoen NL, et al. Acute antibody-mediated rejection of cardiac transplants. Journal of Heart and Lung Transplantation. 2006;**25**:153-159

[54] Becker LE, Morath C, Suesal C. Immune mechanisms of acute and chronic rejection. Clinical Biochemistry. 2016;**49**(4-5):320-323

[55] Weil R 3rd, Clarke DR, Iwaki Y, Porter KA, Koep LJ, Paton BC, et al. Hyperacute rejection of a transplanted human heart. Transplantation. Jul 1981;**32**(1):71-72. PMID: 7022801; PMCID: PMC2964087

[56] Villa C, Mesa K, Cristy Smith M, Mooney DM, Coletti A, Klohe E. Hyperacute graft dysfunction in an orthotopic heart transplant in the presence of non-HLA antibodies. American Journal of Transplantation. 2020;**20**(2):593-599

[57] See Hoe LE, Li Bassi G, Wildi K, Passmore MR, Bouquet M, Sato K, et al. Donor heart ischemic time can be extended beyond 9 hours using hypothermic machine perfusion in sheep. Journal of Heart and Lung Transplantation. 2023;**42**(8):1015-1029

[58] Tang PC, Wu X, Zhang M, Likosky D, Haft JW, Lei I, et al. Determining optimal donor heart ischemic times in adult cardiac transplantation. Journal of Cardiac Surgery. 2022;**37**(7):2042-2050

[59] Santise G, Panarello G, Ruperto C, Turrisi M, Pilato G, Giunta A, et al. Extracorporeal membrane oxygenation for graft failure after heart transplantation: A multidisciplinary approach to maximize weaning rate. International Journal of Artificial Organs. 2014;**37**(9):706-714

[60] Iyer A, Kumarasinghe G, Hicks M, Watson A, Gao L, Doyle A, et al. Primary graft failure after heart transplantation. Journal of Transplantation. 2011;**2011**: 1-9. Available from: http://www.hindawi.com/journals/jtrans/2011/175768/

[61] Chou NK, Chi NH, Ko WJ, Yu HY, Huang SC, Wang SS, et al. Extracorporeal membrane oxygenation for perioperative cardiac allograft failure. ASAIO Journal. 2006;**52**(1):100-103

[62] Frazier EA, Faulkner SC, Seib PM, Harrell JE, Van Devanter SH, Fasules JW. Prolonged Extracorporeal Life Support for Bridging to Transplant: Technical and Mechanical Considerations. Perfusion. Mar 1997;**12**(2):93-98. DOI: 10.1177/026765919701200203. PMID: 9160359

[63] Soleimani B, Pae WE. Management of left ventricular distension during peripheral extracorporeal membrane oxygenation for cardiogenic shock. Perfusion (United Kingdom). 2012;**27**(4):326-331

[64] Lorusso R, Shekar K, MacLaren G, Schmidt M, Pellegrino V, Meyns B, et al. ELSO interim guidelines for venoarterial extracorporeal membrane oxygenation in adult cardiac patients. ASAIO Journal. Lippincott Williams and Wilkins. 2021;**67**:827-844

Chapter 4

Exploring Standard and Alternative Sites for Left Ventricular Assist Device Inflow Cannula and Outflow Graft Placement

Kamen Dimitrov and Daniel Zimpfer

Abstract

Left ventricular assist device (LVAD) therapy is an essential tool in the armamentarium for managing refractory heart failure. The traditional LVAD placement involves insertion of the inflow cannula (IC) at the left ventricle's true apex and attachment of the outflow graft (OG) to the ascending aorta (AA), which ensures alignment with physiological blood flow and minimizes complications. However, patient-specific anatomical variations and prior medical interventions necessitate considering alternative IC and OG placement techniques. This chapter reviews the standard and alternative IC and OG placement sites and emphasizes the importance of adapting LVAD component placement to individual patient needs, highlighting the potential of alternative techniques in improving outcomes. Despite the predominance of standard sites due to their proven efficacy, the heterogeneity of patient conditions underscores the need for flexible, patient-tailored approaches.

Keywords: LVAD, left ventricular assist device, inflow cannula, outflow graft, alternative sites

1. Introduction

Implantable left ventricular assist devices (LVADs) have become an integral part of the therapeutic arsenal for managing end-stage heart failure [1, 2]. Whether serving as a bridge to transplantation or as a long-term solution, the success of these devices is critically dependent on the appropriate placement of their components, primarily the inflow cannula and the outflow graft. This chapter reviews the standard and alternative placement sites for these vital components of contemporary continuous-flow LVADs.

2. Standard and alternative inflow cannula placement

The LVAD relies on three principal blood-contacting components to function: the inflow cannula (IC) – which draws blood from the left side of the heart; the pump – which propels the blood; and the outflow graft (OG) – which returns the blood to the systemic circulation [3, 4]. The placement and position of the IC, however, are crucial considerations for ensuring proper LVAD function, optimal cardiac support, and patient outcomes [3, 5–9]. The left ventricle's (LV) true apex has historically been considered the best placement position of the LVAD's IC and is, therefore, standard [1, 5, 10] (**Table 1**). Several factors rationalize this: IC's placement through the true apex ensures reproducible surgical placement technique. While there may be anatomical variations among patients, the true apex remains a consistently identifiable anatomical landmark [1, 5, 10]. Given its pointed structure and relative anatomical isolation, the LV apex allows for straightforward insertion and secure cannula anchoring. The area is also less prone to hypertrophy, providing a consistent myocardial texture for cannula insertion. From a hemodynamic standpoint, using the true apex as an IC placement entry point ensures the IC's physiological orientation, aligning it with the direction of the physiological blood flow towards the apex [6, 7]. This facilitates more direct flow from the mitral valve to the IC, enhances the device's efficiency, and minimizes blood stasis [6, 8]. The IC must point towards the mitral valve [7] so that its long axis matches the long axis (natural flow axis) of the LV, ensuring that the inflow cannula's orientation is in synchrony with the LV's natural flow trajectory [10, 11]. It also facilitates the direction of the IC that best accommodates the anticipated reductions in LV chamber size occurring over time [8]. Angulation of the IC off-axis towards the interventricular septum or left ventricular free wall may cause intermittent partial occlusion of the IC and suction events, which may lead to poor flow into the LVAD with consequent poor ventricular unloading

Summary of the insertion technique	Advantages	Disadvantages	Contraindications/ Unsuitability	Reasons for unsuitability
Technique of left ventricular assist device (LVAD) implantation that involves direct insertion of the inflow cannula (IC) into the true apex of the left ventricle (LV) via Surgical access: full median sternotomy or lateral thoracotomy or lateral thoracotomy combined with upper hemisternotomy	Well-established with proven outcomes Facilitates standardized LVAD placement Facilitates optimal blood flow from the left ventricle into the LVAD Reduces the risk of inflow obstruction/ suction by adjacent structures.	Potential for ventricular arrhythmias due to manipulation or irritation at the apical site. Risk of inflow cannula malposition due to cardiac remodeling over time. Loss of viable myocardium due at the site of IC placement	Extensive recent myocardial infarction involving the left ventricular apex Extensive myocardial calcifications or thinning at the apex Previous apical surgeries or interventions that have altered the LV anatomy	Extensive myocardial scarring or thinning can result in inadequate or unstable cannula fixation, increasing the risk of complications such as bleeding or device malfunction. Previous surgical interventions can present anatomical challenges or increase risks.

Table 1.
Left ventricular assist device implantation with inflow cannula placement at the true apex.

and possible hemolysis or thromboembolic complications [3, 6–9]. The standard IC placement technique - ensuring that the IC's orientation aligns with the direction of physiological blood flow towards the apex, facilitating direct flow from the mitral valve to the IC -should therefore reduce the risk of inflow obstruction, suction events, and thrombosis that can lead to ventricular arrhythmias or device alarms and stroke [7, 9]. Numerical (in silico) and clinical data support the adverse effects of off-axis angulation of the IC [7, 9, 11–13]. The attachment of the IC to the myocardium is facilitated by a sewing ring that is attached to the epicardial surface near the LV's true apex, usually at its anterior wall, about 2 cm lateral to the left anterior descending coronary artery [1, 5, 10]. A circular knife creates a myocardial core directed towards the mitral valve and parallel to the interventricular septum [14]. Different IC surgical fixation techniques exist [15]. In this regard, in in-vitro studies, the sew-then-core technique using epicardial stitching, in which partial-thickness suture bites do not penetrate the endocardium, appears to be associated with the lowest risk of suction events or thrombosis formation [15]. Although lacking robustness, available clinical data has indeed shown a trend towards a higher risk of stroke when the cut-then-sew" technique is utilized compared to the "cut-then-sew" approach [16]. Future studies should also confirm whether surgical access techniques (lateral thoracotomy versus conventional full sternotomy) play a role in optimal IC positioning [12].

The choice of the apical site for IC has been supported by decades of clinical experience. However, it is crucial to consider the individual patient's anatomy, comorbidities, and potential for complications when opting for the standard site [1, 10]. In this regard, several clinical scenarios, such as previous cardiac surgery, severe apical calcifications, aneurismal dilation or thinning of the apical wall, apical hypertrophy, or unique anatomical variations may make apical IC placement unpractical, risky, or undesirable [1, 5, 10, 17] (**Table 2**). These special situations might require exploring

Summary of the insertion technique	Advantages	Disadvantages	Contraindications/ Unsuitability	Reasons for unsuitability
Technique of left ventricular assist device (LVAD) implantation that involves placing the inflow cannula at a site other than the standard apical location (e.g., left atrium, left ventricular basal wall, in a patch used for LV reconstruction (Dor procedure)). Surgical access: full median sternotomy.	Addresses patient-specific anatomical challenges and facilitates optimal IC positioning and LVAD function (significant LV hypertrophy/ small LV cavity, apical aneurism with/without thrombus formation)	Increased operative complexity/ technical challenges	Cases suitable for IC placement into the true apex IC placement in the lateral LV free wall	IC placement in the lateral LV free wall could increase the risk of suboptimal IC position, suction events and suboptimal LVAD function

Table 2.
Left ventricular assist device implantation with alternative inflow cannula placement.

unconventional IC placement sites with a certain degree of surgical flexibility and innovation [10], tailored to serve patient's needs best [1, 5, 10]. A recent extensive myocardial necrosis involving the apex may also preclude safe anchoring of the IC's sewing ring. In this case, the IC's sewing ring may be attached to a Dacron patch used to reconstruct the excised necrotic apex [18]. That can also be applied in the cases of concomitant left ventricular reconstruction for (severely calcified) ventricular aneurism or a previous Dor procedure [10, 19–22]. Cannulation of the left ventricular diaphragmatic wall may be a viable alternative to this [1, 10]. Attachment of the IC to the diaphragmatic wall may also be useful in cases of a markedly enlarged LV with altered geometry, the presence of post-myocardial infarction apical aneurysm, and patients with constricted thoracic anatomy [1, 5, 10]. Next, with a significant representation of about 2% among LVAD recipients, patients with restrictive or hypertrophic cardiomyopathy are more prone to right ventricular failure, suction events, and death during LVAD support [23, 24]. The adverse outcomes observed in this specific fraction of LVAD patients are likely due to their distinctive anatomy – having small left ventricular cavities [23, 24] and making them ineligible or challenging for standard apical cannulation [23, 25, 26]. In these cases, a myectomy may be necessary so that enough space is created for the IC [25]. Alternatively, atrial cannulation can be performed, especially considering considerable left atrial enlargement in this patient population [23]. A novel transseptal technique has been described, in which the IC is connected to the left atrium through a Gore-Tex® tube placed into the right atrium and sewn to the surgically created interatrial septum defect [23, 27]. In this case, the sewing ring is attached to the right atrium and the interposition graft [23, 28].

Ultimately, a novel technique intending to overcome the risks associated with the development of intracavitary clot formation and its sequelae has been proposed, in which the IC is attached to a cone-shaped prosthesis connecting the left ventricular apex with the mitral valve [29].

Conclusively, while the true apex of the LV remains the standard and most widely used site for IC placement, the vast array of individual patient anatomies, previous medical interventions, and unique conditions dictate the necessity for adaptable and innovative approaches, guided by the overriding principles of ensuring the best possible outcomes for the patient.

3. Standard and alternative outflow graft placement

The outflow graft is attached to the ascending aorta (AA) in an end-to-side fashion, facilitating blood flow from the LVAD to the systemic circulation, and is considered the standard practice in most LVAD implantations [1, 5, 10]. The recommended and preferred anastomosis site at the AA is at its right concavity, about 2 cm above the sinotubular junction [1, 10] (**Table 3**). In patients with an untouched pericardium (no previous pericardiotomy) for instance, the recommended course of the OG should be intrapericardial, along the inferior right ventricular surface and between the right atrium and pericardium so that the right ventricular outflow tract remains uncrossed [1]. Optionally, tunneling the outflow graft through the transverse sinus with OG anastomosis at the posterolateral aspect of the AA may also be considered [1]. Ultimately, while still preferably connecting it to the AA, routing the OG within the left pleural cavity may also be considered to reduce operative complexity in redo procedures [1].

Summary of the insertion technique	Advantages	Disadvantages	Contraindications/ Unsuitability	Reasons for unsuitability
Technique of left ventricular assist device (LVAD) implantation involving anastomosing the outflow graft (OG) to the ascending aorta (AA). Surgical access: full median sternotomy or less invasive (a lateral thoracotomy combined with an upper hemisternotomy or bilateral thoracotomy) with routing of the OG between the right atrium and the pericardium or the transverse sinus.	Well-established with proven outcomes Facilitates standardized LVAD placement Direct flow into the aorta Reduced risk of OG kinking or obstruction	Requires mediastinal (re-) entry/surgical exposure of the AA Risk of complications in patients with severe atherosclerosis of the AA a "hostile chest" (previous cardiac surgery/ mediastinal radiation leading to mediastinal scarring/ adhesions/ severe chest wall deformities	Severe atherosclerosis of the AA "Hostile chest" (previous cardiac surgery/mediastinal radiation leading to mediastinal scarring/adhesions/ severe chest wall deformities	Increased risk of embolism/stroke/ aortic dissection in cases of severe atherosclerosis of the AA Limited surgical access and increased surgical complexity due to mediastinal adhesions/patent coronary artery bypass grafts/ severe chest wall deformities. Risk of inadvertent damage to mediastinal structures due to severe mediastinal adhesions Risk of inadvertent damage to patent coronary artery bypass grafts

Table 3.
Left ventricular assist device implantation with outflow graft placement to the ascending aorta.

The ascending aorta is a central conduit in the systemic circulation, making it a logical point to introduce blood pumped by the LVAD to be distributed throughout the body. Attaching the OG to the AA is favored because of the AA's large diameter, good anatomical accessibility, the relative ease with which the anastomosis is completed, postulated in decades of clinical experience. Besides the precise positioning of the IC, however, optimal LVAD performance is equally contingent upon the rigorous positioning of the outflow graft. Traditionally, the AA is the gold standard for OG anastomosis, capitalizing on its central position in the systemic circulation and its presumably resilient anatomy to withstand long-term pressure and flow conditions impaired by the LVAD. That said, the proximal aorta does undergoes dilation under LVAD support [30]. This, on the other side, has been correlated to the development of de novo aortic valve regurgitation, which is more likely to occur in patients with preexisting (before LVAD implant) aortic dilation [30, 31]. These alterations are presumably the results of the LVAD support-induced unphysiological hemodynamics [30, 31]. In this regard, the results of computational fluid dynamics studies confidently advocate for positioning the OG so that it directs the jet of blood towards the lumen of the aortic arch, aiming to prevent turbulent flow, subsequently reducing wall stress and backward pressure in the aortic root [32]. Both in-silico studies and existing clinical data have confirmed that any deviation of the LVAD outflow jet from the normal flow direction in the AA can lead to flow stasis, aortic root thrombosis, and thromboembolic complications [33–36]. Indeed, a 45° angulation of the outflow graft-to-ascending aorta anastomosis to reduce the risk of de novo aortic valve regurgitation during LVAD support is currently recommended by experts in the field [1]. Nevertheless, the optimal orientation of the OG anastomosis, as well as its distance from the aortic root, are yet to be established in future research [32].

Further, just as the LV's anatomy and function govern the complexities of the inflow cannula's positioning, it is crucial to consider the individual patient's anatomy, comorbid conditions, and potential for complications – and all that in the context of the surgeon's expertise when opting for placement of the OG anastomosis to the standard site. An improperly placed OG might impede natural blood flow, potentially leading to complications such as graft occlusion, turbulent blood flow, or even damage to the aorta itself. Besides that, OG anastomosis to the AA may be nonamenable in patients with hostile chest anatomy or porcelain aorta [1, 10]. Anatomical variations (i.e., severe aortic calcifications, severe chest wall deformities, presence of patent grafts from prior coronary artery bypass surgery, previous AA procedures) or presence of extensive mediastinal adhesions (e.g., post radiation therapy or prior previous cardiac surgery) may deem the surgical access or placement of the OG anastomosis at the AA challenging, high-risk or even prohibitively hazardous, even in experienced hands. To specifically address this, surgical LVAD implantation techniques involving alternative OG landing sites have been developed [1, 10, 37] (**Figure 1**, **Table 4**). Several surgical techniques involving OG placement to the innominate artery, axillary/subclavian artery, descending aorta, or supra-celiac abdominal aorta have been described [4, 32]. While these unconventional sites may offer certain benefits resulting from the less invasive operative technique, like the potentially reduced operative exposure, the use of blood products, the incidence of right heart failure, or avoiding sternotomy in redo surgeries, they come with challenges, including ensuring proper graft orientation and strategies to prevent kinking of the OG and increased operative complexity [10, 38, 39]. In this line of thought, the seemingly indispensable reinforcement of the OG using a (ringed) vascular graft protector has been associated with the development of the unique late complication - OG stenosis, in some patients [40, 41]. Moreover, minimally invasive approaches for LVAD implantation with OG anastomosis to the AA have been standardized, and their benefits are well described [38, 42–44].

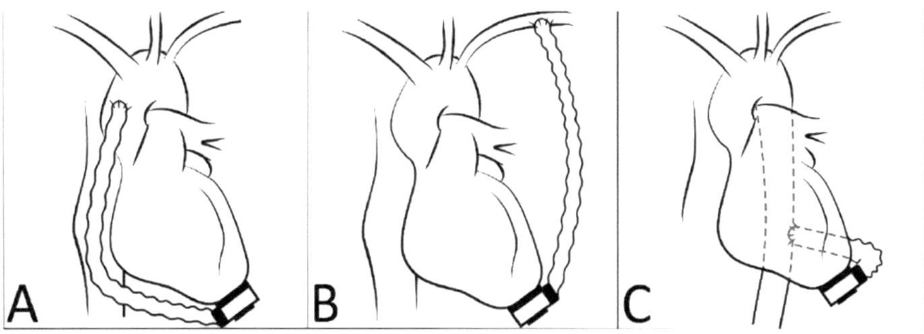

Figure 1.
Standard and alternative outflow graft anastomosis sites. Schematic depiction of left ventricular assist device placed onto the left ventricular apex with outflow graft anastomosis to the ascending aorta (A), subclavian/axillary artery (B) and descending aorta (C).

Summary of the insertion technique	Advantages	Disadvantages	Contraindications/ Unsuitability	Reasons for unsuitability
Technique of left ventricular assist device (LVAD) implantation involving OG placement to the innominate artery, axillary/ subclavian artery, descending aorta, or supra-celiac abdominal aorta. Surgical access: less-invasive sternotomy-sparing approaches (lateral thoracotomy (thoracotomies), or thoracotomy combined with an upper abdominal incision, depending on the chosen anastomosis site).	Useful in cases of a "hostile chest" or severe atherosclerosis/ calcifications to the ascending aorta Preservation of a virgin mediastinum	Challenges in graft routing to prevent OG kinking or twisting Limited target vessel diameter for OG anastomosis Risk of arm hyperperfusion/ swelling Limited data on long-term outcomes and clinical consequences of a retrograde flow systemic perfusion and altered "washout" of the aortic root and ascending aorta	Significant atherosclerosis at the anastomosis site Coarctation of the aorta/severe atherosclerotic obstruction proximal to the anastomosis Small-caliber vessel for the distal OG anastomosis	Significant atherosclerosis at the anastomosis site may increase the risk of vascular dissection/ embolization. Coarctation can impact flow dynamics, affecting LVAD function and patient hemodynamics. A too small vessel diameter might not allow for optimal (LVAD) blood flow or may complicate the anastomosis procedure.

Table 4.
Left ventricular assist device implantation with alternative outflow anastomosis sites.

Yet, LVAD placement with OG to the left axillary/subclavian artery or descending aorta offers one more advantage, that is, "the preservation of a virgin chest" in patients who are deemed transplant candidates [39, 45]. However, the clinically significant hemodynamic sequelae and long-term outcomes associated with these alternative OG locations are unknown [39, 46], and they are therefore to be regarded as valid but not equal alternatives to the standard OG location [1, 39].

In the end, the choice of OG placement should be determined by a combination of the patient's unique anatomy, clinical history, and the surgeon's expertise, always with an eye on ensuring the longevity and efficiency of the LVAD system.

4. Conclusion

While LVAD technology and surgical techniques continue to evolve, the standard sites for inflow and outflow component placement remain prevalent due to their ease of access, reduced surgical complexity, and favorable long-term outcomes. Nevertheless, ongoing research and clinical experience continue to inform best practices, suggesting that what is considered "standard" today may be subject to change in the light of new evidence.

5. Discussion

Implantable LVADs have revolutionized the treatment of end-stage heart failure [2, 47]. The placement of the IC into the true LV apex and the OG at the ascending aorta have become standards in LVAD implantation techniques with implications in ways that go beyond simple surgical convenience - the optimal positioning of these components has a significant impact on patient outcomes and the efficiency of the LVAD system [1, 2, 47, 48]. However, modifications to the standard surgical techniques of IC and OG placement exploiting their different landing sites and attachment methods can be made to address particular patient demands [10]. Such alternative techniques might also gain popularity as our knowledge of the dynamics and physiology of heart failure advances, and new technical advancements take hold. Moreover, avoiding access to the ascending aorta in the cases of alternative OG placement techniques offers the convenience of a quasi-virgin mediastinum, which should ease future reoperation and improve outcomes in heart transplant recipients [39, 45, 49]. Big, granular data on long-term outcomes with alternative IC and OG placement techniques is not available yet, and standard implantation sites remain predominant in clinical practice due to their proven efficacy, as evidenced by decades of clinical experience [1]. Nevertheless, the vast heterogeneity of patient conditions and clinical scenarios necessitates the consideration of alternative and unconventional approaches to device placement, which provide invaluable solutions in situations when patient-specific variables prevent routine implantation [1, 10, 37]. These approaches are not merely alternatives, but often tailored strategies devised in the face of challenges that the standard practices cannot address.

Further detailed research assessing the standard and alternative LVAD implantation techniques should provide insights that facilitate further refinements in these approaches that translate into improvements in patient outcomes. As the field continues to advance, it is paramount to prioritize patient-specific considerations while pursuing optimization, durability, and safety.

Acknowledgements

We are thankful to Alica Dimitrova for the design of **Figure 1**.

Conflict of interest

The authors declare no conflict of interest.

Author details

Kamen Dimitrov* and Daniel Zimpfer
Department of Cardiac Surgery, Medical University of Vienna, Vienna, Austria

*Address all correspondence to: kamen.dimitrov@meduniwien.ac.at

References

[1] Potapov EV, Antonides C, Crespo-Leiro MG, Combes A, Färber G, Hannan MM, et al. 2019 EACTS expert consensus on long-term mechanical circulatory support. European Journal of Cardio-Thoracic Surgery. 2019;**56**(2):230-270

[2] McDonagh TA, Metra M, Adamo M, Gardner RS, Baumbach A, Böhm M, et al. 2021 ESC Guidelines for the diagnosis and treatment of acute and chronic heart failure: Developed by the Task Force for the diagnosis and treatment of acute and chronic heart failure of the European Society of Cardiology (ESC) with the special contribution of the Heart Failure Association (HFA) of the ESC. European Heart Journal. 2021;**42**(36):3599-3726

[3] Gopinathannair R, Cornwell WK, Dukes JW, Ellis CR, Hickey KT, Joglar JA, et al. Device therapy and arrhythmia management in left ventricular assist device recipients: A scientific statement from the American Heart Association. Circulation. 2019;**139**(20):e967-ee89

[4] Miller L, Birks E, Guglin M, Lamba H, Frazier OH. Use of ventricular assist devices and heart transplantation for advanced heart failure. Circulation Research. 2019;**124**(11):1658-1678

[5] Kirklin JK, Pagani FD, Goldstein DJ, John R, Rogers JG, Atluri P, et al. American Association for Thoracic Surgery/International Society for Heart and Lung Transplantation guidelines on selected topics in mechanical circulatory support. The Journal of Heart and Lung Transplantation. 2020;**39**(3):187-219

[6] Maraouch G, Kadem L. Flow dynamics in a model of a left ventricle with different mitral valve orientations. Fluids. 2021;**6**(12):428

[7] Neidlin M, Liao S, Li Z, Simpson B, Kaye DM, Steinseifer U, et al. Understanding the influence of left ventricular assist device inflow cannula alignment and the risk of intraventricular thrombosis. BioMedical Engineering OnLine. 2021;**20**(1):47

[8] Slaughter MS, Pagani FD, Rogers JG, Miller LW, Sun B, Russell SD, et al. Clinical management of continuous-flow left ventricular assist devices in advanced heart failure. The Journal of Heart and Lung Transplantation. 2010;**29**(4, Supplement):S1-S39

[9] Chivukula VK, Beckman JA, Li S, Masri SC, Levy WC, Lin S, et al. Left ventricular assist device inflow cannula insertion depth influences thrombosis risk. ASAIO Journal. 2020;**66**(7)

[10] Loforte A, Bottio T, Attisani M, Suarez SM, Tarzia V, Pocar M, et al. Conventional and alternative sites for left ventricular assist device inflow and outflow cannula placement. Annals of Cardiothoracic Surgery. 2021;**10**(2):281-288

[11] Kortekaas KA, de Graaf MA, Palmen M, Braun J, Mertens BJA, Tops LF, et al. Left ventricular assist device and pump thrombosis: The importance of the inflow cannula position. The International Journal of Cardiovascular Imaging. 2022;**38**(12):2771-2779

[12] Schlöglhofer T, Aigner P, Migas M, Beitzke D, Wittmann F, Riebandt J, et al. Inflow cannula position as predictor for neurological dysfunction in patients with HeartMate 3 left ventricular assist device. The Journal of Heart and Lung Transplantation. 2020;**39**(4):S97-SS8

[13] Schlöglhofer T, Aigner P, Migas M, Beitzke D, Dimitrov K, Wittmann F, et al. Inflow cannula position as risk factor for stroke in patients with HeartMate 3 left ventricular assist devices. Artificial Organs. 2022;**46**(6):1149-1157

[14] Netuka I. HeartMate 3 left ventricular assist system implantation technique: The devil is in the detail†. Interactive CardioVascular and Thoracic Surgery. 2018;**27**(6):946-949

[15] Hanke JS, Krabatsch T, Rojas SV, Deniz E, Ismail I, Martens A, et al. In vitro evaluation of inflow cannula fixation techniques in left ventricular assist device surgery. Artificial Organs. 2017;**41**:272-275

[16] Salerno C, Naka Y, Silvestry SC, Goldstein DJ, Cleveland JC, Bansal A, et al. HeartMate 3 surgical implant technique and outcomes in the MOMENTUM 3 Trial. The Journal of Heart and Lung Transplantation. 2019;**38**(4, Supplement):S78

[17] Di Stefano S, Sarralde JA, San Román JA, Stepanenko A. Challenges in cannulation of left ventricular apex for temporary circulatory support: A case report. AME Case Report. 2021;**5**:32

[18] Marasco SF, McDonald C, McGiffin DC. Chapter 15 - surgical implantation. In: Gregory SD, Stevens MC, Fraser JF, editors. Mechanical Circulatory and Respiratory Support. Academic Press; 2018. pp. 469-494

[19] Piperata A, Kalscheuer G, Pernot M, Albadi W, Metras A, Peltan J, et al. Left ventricle reconstruction and heartmate3 implantation. The 'double patch technique'. Journal of Cardiac Surgery. 2020;**35**(11):3116-3119

[20] Osaki S, Edwards NM, Kohmoto T. Strategies for left ventricular assist device insertion after the Dor procedure. The Journal of Heart and Lung Transplantation. 2009;**28**(5):520-522

[21] Smith JW, Pal JD, Walters D, Mahr CM, Mokadam NA. Left ventricular assist device placement with concomitant ventricular reconstruction for aneurysmal disease. The Journal of Heart and Lung Transplantation. 2016;**35**(4):S372

[22] Gyoten T, Ono M. Outcomes of continuous flow left ventricular assist device after surgical left ventricular restoration. General Thoracic and Cardiovascular Surgery. 2023;**71**(8):480-486

[23] Kiamanesh O, Rankin K, Billia F, Badiwala MV. Left ventricular assist device with a left atrial inflow cannula for hypertrophic cardiomyopathy. JACC: Case Reports. 2020;**2**(13):2090-2094

[24] Sreenivasan J, Kaul R, Khan MS, Ranka S, Demmer RT, Yuzefpolskaya M, et al. Left ventricular assist device implantation in hypertrophic and restrictive cardiomyopathy: A systematic review. ASAIO Journal. 2021;**67**(3)

[25] Topilsky Y, Pereira NL, Shah DK, Boilson B, Schirger JA, Kushwaha SS, et al. Left ventricular assist device therapy in patients with restrictive and hypertrophic cardiomyopathy. Circulation: Heart Failure. 2011;**4**(3):266-275

[26] Grupper A, Park SJ, Pereira NL, Schettle SD, Gerber Y, Topilsky Y, et al. Role of ventricular assist therapy for patients with heart failure and restrictive physiology: Improving outcomes for a lethal disease. The Journal of Heart and Lung Transplantation. 2015;**34**(8):1042-1049

[27] Maeda K, Nasirov T, Yarlagadda V, Hollander SA,

Navarathnum M, Rosenthal DN, et al. Novel trans-septal left atrial VAD cannulation technique for hypertrophic/ restrictive cardiomyopathy. The Journal of Heart and Lung Transplantation. 2019;**38**(4, Supplement):S479

[28] Lim CP, Lim YP, Lim CH, Ong H-Y, Tan D, Omar AR. Two-year outcome of ventricular assist device via a modified left atrium to aorta approach in cardiac amyloidosis. ESC Heart Failure. 2022;**9**(5):3597-3601

[29] Klotz S, Meyer-Saraei R, Frydrychowicz A, Scharfschwerdt M, Putman LM, Halder S, et al. Proposing a novel technique to exclude the left ventricle with an assist device: Insights from 4-dimensional flow magnetic resonance imaging †. European Journal of Cardio-Thoracic Surgery. 2016;**50**(3):439-445

[30] Fine NM, Park SJ, Stulak JM, Topilsky Y, Daly RC, Joyce LD, et al. Proximal thoracic aorta dimensions after continuous-flow left ventricular assist device implantation: Longitudinal changes and relation to aortic valve insufficiency. The Journal of Heart and Lung Transplantation. 2016;**35**(4):423-432

[31] Nishida H, Song T, Onsager D, Nguyen A, Grinstein J, Chung B, et al. Proximal ascending aorta size is associated with the incidence of de novo aortic insufficiency with left ventricular assist device. Heart and Vessels. 2022;**37**(4):647-653

[32] Karmonik C, Partovi S, Loebe M, Schmack B, Weymann A, Lumsden AB, et al. Computational fluid dynamics in patients with continuous-flow left ventricular assist device support show hemodynamic alterations in the ascending aorta. The Journal of Thoracic and Cardiovascular Surgery. 2014;**147**(4):1326

[33] Kassi M, Karmonik C, Engelke J, Eshelbrenner C, Rehman H, Belousova T, et al. Correlation of LVAD outflow graft orientation with aortic root thrombosis rationalized by patient specific computational fluid dynamics simulations. The Journal of Heart and Lung Transplantation. 2016;**35**(4):S246

[34] Aliseda A, Chivukula VK, McGah P, Prisco AR, Beckman JA, Garcia GJ, et al. LVAD outflow graft angle and thrombosis risk. ASAIO Journal. 2017;**63**(1):14-23

[35] Sahni A, McIntyre EE, Pal JD, Mukherjee D. Quantitative assessment of aortic Hemodynamics for varying left ventricular assist device outflow graft angles and flow pulsation. Annals of Biomedical Engineering. 2023;**51**(6):1226-1243

[36] Peek JJ, Zijderhand C, Sjatskig J, van der Heiden C, Constantinescu AA, Brugts JJ, et al. (125) Influence of the outflow graft position on thromboembolic and bleeding complications in patients with a left ventricular assist device. The Journal of Heart and Lung Transplantation. 2023;**42**(4, Supplement):S65

[37] El-Sayed Ahmed MM, Aftab M, Singh SK, Mallidi HR, Frazier OH. Left ventricular assist device outflow graft: Alternative sites. Annals of Cardiothoracic Surgery. 2014;**3**(5):541-545

[38] Haberl T, Riebandt J, Mahr S, Laufer G, Rajek A, Schima H, et al. Viennese approach to minimize the invasiveness of ventricular assist device implantation†. European Journal of Cardio-Thoracic Surgery. 2014;**46**(6):991-996 discussion 6

[39] Nguyen SN, Nguyen TC. Commentary: Less-invasive approaches to big complex problems in patients

with end-stage heart disease. JTCVS Techniques. 2020;**4**:200-201

[40] Dimitrov K, Kaider A, Angleitner P, Schlöglhofer T, Gross C, Beitzke D, et al. Incidence, clinical relevance and therapeutic options for outflow graft stenosis in patients with left ventricular assist devices. European Journal of Cardio-Thoracic Surgery. 2022;**61**(3):716-724

[41] Dimitrov K, Kaider A, Granegger M, Gross C, Angleitner P, Wiedemann D, et al. The effect of occlusive polytetrafluoroethylene outflow graft protectors in left ventricular assist device recipients. The Journal of Heart and Lung Transplantation. 2022;**41**(12):1850-1857

[42] Carmona A, Hoang Minh T, Perrier S, Schneider C, Marguerite S, Ajob G, et al. Minimally invasive surgery for left ventricular assist device implantation is safe and associated with a decreased risk of right ventricular failure. Journal of Thoracic Disease. 2020;**12**(4):1496-1506

[43] Reineke DC, Carrel TP. Less invasive left ventricular assist device implantation-a match changer! Journal of Thoracic Disease. 2015;**7**(5):783-786

[44] Riebandt J, Schlöglhofer T, Moayedifar R, Wiedemann D, Wittmann F, Angleitner P, et al. Less invasive left ventricular assist device implantation is safe and reduces intraoperative blood product use: A propensity score analysis VAD implantation techniques and blood product use. ASAIO Journal. 2021;**67**(1):47-52

[45] Riebandt J, Wiedemann D, Sandner S, Angleitner P, Zuckermann A, Schlöglhofer T, et al. Impact of less invasive left ventricular assist device implantation on heart transplant outcomes. Seminars in Thoracic and Cardiovascular Surgery. 2022;**34**(1):148-156

[46] Caruso MV, Gramigna V, Rossi M, Serraino GF, Renzulli A, Fragomeni G. A computational fluid dynamics comparison between different outflow graft anastomosis locations of left ventricular assist device (LVAD) in a patient-specific aortic model. International Journal for Numerical Methods in Biomedical Engineering. 2015;**31**(2):e02700

[47] Yuzefpolskaya M, Schroeder SE, Houston BA, Robinson MR, Gosev I, Reyentovich A, et al. The Society of Thoracic Surgeons Intermacs 2022 annual report: Focus on the 2018 heart transplant allocation system. The Annals of Thoracic Surgery. 2023;**115**(2):311-327

[48] Imamura T, Nguyen A, Chung B, Rodgers D, Sarswat N, Kim G, et al. Association of Inflow Cannula Position with left ventricular unloading and clinical outcomes in patients with HeartMate II left ventricular assist device. ASAIO Journal. 2019;**65**(4):331-335

[49] Ribeiro RVP, Alvarez JS, Fukunaga N, Yu F, Adamson MB, Foroutan F, et al. Redo sternotomy versus left ventricular assist device explant as risk factors for early mortality following heart transplantation. Interactive CardioVascular and Thoracic Surgery. 2020;**31**(5):603-610

Chapter 5

LVAD Continuing Care: A Comprehensive Guide to Long-Term Support and Management

Michael Sobieraj, Brisha Bhikadiya-Best, Sabaa Ahmed, Stephen Crawford and Kulpreet Barn

Abstract

Heart failure is a growing pandemic with a rising societal burden. Heart failure affects 3.6 million people in Europe and 5 million in the United States annually. The United States alone spends 30.7 billion annually managing heart failure, and that number is expected to eclipse 70 billion by 2030. Many people are not orthotopic heart transplant candidates, and many who are may not live long enough to receive a transplant. As a result, durable left ventricular assist devices (LVAD) have become both a bridging therapy and a destination therapy, necessitating a robust continuing care system. LVAD programs are expanding to fill this need. This chapter aims to cover the spectrum of LVAD continuing care from initial implantation to the outpatient clinic. This chapter will cover essential care practices for maintaining LVAD function, including driveline care, battery management, and alarm response/tracking. Troubleshooting the common issues and complications patients might experience, such as low flow alarms, bleeding, infection, and right heart failure. Emphasize the importance of the primary caregiver's involvement and how to prepare them by providing resources for education, training, and ongoing support. Lastly, it will cover ethical concerns and the role of palliative care in the process.

Keywords: LVAD, left ventricular assist device, advanced heart failure, advanced therapies, durable mechanical circulatory support, durable LVAD, end stage heart failure

1. Introduction

Heart failure (HF) is a global pandemic that has been increasing in prevalence. It affects 3.6 million people in Europe and 5 million in the United States (US) annually. Left ventricular assist devices (LVADs) were first introduced as a bridge to orthotopic heart transplant (OHT) and subsequently progressed into a viable long-term therapeutic option [1]. With prevalence now approaching 2% in the US and Canada and hospitalization rates as high as 3%, it comes as no surprise that $30.7 billion was spent annually in the US alone managing this critical diagnosis. Further, the cost is expected to exceed $70 billion by 2030 [2, 3].

Varying stages of HF come with progressively more severe disability for the patient and a progressively increasing need for more social support. End-stage heart failure leads to significantly higher morbidity with loss of autonomy and increasing societal costs [4]. OHT remains the gold standard for end-stage HF as it still boasts the most longevity when there is a favorable surgical outcome. Due to the limited availability of organs, many contraindications limit the eligible recipient pool greatly. Some of these include age greater than 70 years, severe pulmonary hypertension, severe lung disease, severe infection, viral infections with organ damage, a history of cancer, severe neurological deficits, psychiatric illness, current tobacco or recreational drug use, multisystem disease with poor long term survival, and many more [5]. For patients who are not ideal OHT candidates, LVAD remains an option, with a mean survival now surpassing 7.1 years [6]. For some patients, LVADs may serve as a bridge to transplantation, while for others it may be a final destination therapy. For those that are not LVAD candidates, those with severe right ventricular failure, restrictive or hypertrophic cardiomyopathy, left ventricular end-diastolic dimension <4.5 cm, or contraindications to anticoagulation, a palliative care referral is indicated [7].

2. Patient selection for LVAD therapy

The population of people living with advanced heart failure is growing along with the need for advanced therapies. From 2006 through 2017, there have been 25,000 durable LVADs implanted [8]. This boost in implantation was largely due to the advent of the superior continuous flow LVADs which tripled the volumes being recorded in the Interagency Registry for Mechanically Assisted Circulatory Support (INTERMACS) registry [8]. Firstly, there are two major LVAD indications that are accepted by both payors and governing bodies in medicine alike, either as a bridge to heart transplant (BTT) or as a final destination therapy (DT) in the setting of refractory end-stage heart failure [8]. It is also worth noting a more recent and controversial indication that is not recognized by the FDA which is being called "bridge to candidacy (BTC)." In this patient population, the LVAD is implanted officially as a DT, however, the heart team is hoping later to improve the patient's candidacy for a heart transplant. One example is an obese patient who would otherwise be a good OHT candidate where the LVAD is implanted with the hope of having the patient improve their BMI through weight management and/or bariatric surgery in order to become an eligible OHT candidate later. The least common implantation indication is as a bridge-to-recovery (BTR). While this remains a rare occurrence, only accounting for less than 3% of all LVAD recipients, there is recent retrospective data demonstrating that 40% of patients with a NICM and duration of HF less than or equal to 5 years at the time of implantation were alive and still not requiring MCS or OHT at 1-year post-LVAD explantation [9]. In the United States, the Centers for Medicaid and Medicare Services officially recognize the terms "short-term" and "long-term" in regard to the intention of LVAD implantation [8]. Patients who do qualify for an LVAD must undergo a qualification process to optimize their success post-surgery [10]. Risk stratification begins by classifying the patient with an INTERMACS profile. INTERMACS profiles range from 1 to 7, with 1 being the most severely decompensated cases of cardiogenic shock that require mechanical circulatory support (MCS) and 7 being the most compensated patients (**Table 1**).

INTERMACS	
1	Life-threatening cardiogenic shock despite inotropic support
2	Declining functional status despite inotropic support
3	Stable on inotropic support
4	Symptoms at rest (NYHA Class IV)
5	Symptoms with activity (NYHA Class III)
6	Symptoms within minutes of activity
7	Living comfortably (NYHA Class II)

Table 1.
INTERMACS profile descriptions.

The advanced heart failure team will typically try to evaluate candidacy while the patient is still in INTERMACS profiles 3–4 where the post-surgical outcomes typically fare better than INTERMACS profiles 1 and 2.

LVAD candidacy evaluation should include a heart failure specialist, cardiac surgeons, anesthesiology, palliative care, psychology, and social work [11]. Additionally, multiple risk factors including the patient's age, renal function, liver function, hyponatremia, pulmonary disease, glucose tolerance, dysrhythmias, functional capacity, and history of recurrent admissions are all assessed [12]. All patients being evaluated for a durable LVAD should have early consultation with a palliative care specialist to establish each individual patient's goals of care by improving symptom management, setting realistic expectations, and clearly defining end-of-life care preferences. Progressive renal dysfunction is associated with a poorer prognosis, so it is generally recommended to implant the LVAD before developing severe cardiorenal syndrome or to place a temporary MCS device and monitor for improvement. For pulmonary assessment, it is recommended that the patient have a baseline chest X-ray and undergo invasive hemodynamic assessment. Routine ABGs are not required and there is limited data to validate the benefit of routine pulmonary function testing, but both may be useful if occult disease, such as COPD, is suspected [13]. CT or MRI to evaluate the chest anatomy in patients with a prior history of cardiac surgery is a reasonable choice pre-implantation for surgical planning. All patients should have a comprehensive neurological physical exam and any significant findings, including dementia and severe neuromuscular disease warrant a neurological consultation as these patients may not be able to manage their equipment. A CT head or an MRI may be considered if there is a prior history of stroke to establish a baseline. All patients should also have peripheral vascular disease screening by carotid and vertebral Doppler examinations. All patients should have their PT, aPTT, and INR checked and if an abnormality is found then it needs to be investigated as thrombophilia could thrombose the LVAD. Patients with a history of cancer in long-term remission may be candidates for DT LVAD. Patients with active malignancy, but a life expectancy greater than 2 years may also be considered for DT LVAD therapy in consultation with an oncologist. DT LVAD is not recommended in patients with an active malignancy and a life expectancy of less than 2 years. All patients should be screened for diabetes and those with known diabetes should have their glycemic control optimized prior to surgery. Women of reproductive age should be screened for pregnancy as durable LVADs are contraindicated during active pregnancy. Endoscopy and colonoscopy are reasonable in patients with a history of gastrointestinal bleeding or premalignant polyps.

Right heart failure (RHF) can be a common post-LVAD implantation complication, therefore the right ventricle must be thoroughly evaluated by a multifaceted approach that incorporates physical exam findings, invasive hemodynamics, echocardiography, and other advanced imaging modalities [14]. The gold standard of RV function and structural assessment is the cardiac MRI. Unfortunately, the utilization of MR may be limited in this population by device incompatibility. Right heart strain and 3D echocardiography have improved the ability to identify right heart failure on echocardiography and may be considered. While there is no ideal individual risk assessment tool for right heart failure, there are several predictive models that may be considered: Michigan RCF, Penn RVAD, Heartmate II bridge-to-transplantation RVF analysis, Utah RVF, Pittsburgh decision tree, EuroMACS, and other similar ones have been noted in the literature [14].

Cardiopulmonary stress testing (CPET) can be useful with peak oxygen consumption levels ≤12 mL/kg/min on beta-blocker therapy or ≤ 14 mL/kg/min off of beta-blocker therapy warranting further evaluation for advanced therapies [15]. Additionally, the patient's home should be evaluated for safety (lack of clutter, grounded electrical outlets, reliable telephone access, and emergency medical service access). The patient's psychosocial status should be assessed to evaluate the patient's capabilities and decision-making capacity as well as to mitigate any barriers to the patient being able to care for them self and manage the device. Psychosocial assessment aids in the success of post-LVAD morbidity and mortality. The Stanford Integrated Psychosocial Assessment for Transplantation (SIPAT) is a tool that can be used to determine post-implantation healthcare needs and behaviors. It analyzes a patient's preparedness, social support system, psychosocial stability, and lifestyle effects [16]. Any patient with a significant psychiatric disorder should be evaluated by a psychiatrist. Patients with a history of tobacco and marijuana use should receive counseling on the importance of cessation. Implanting centers vary on their respective policies in regard to marijuana use given the changing legal climate. Patients with a history of alcohol or other substance abuse must be abstinent for a period of time determined by the implanting centers. Active users of alcohol or other substance abuse should not receive an LVAD. The presence of a caregiver and their ability to participate in equipment and driveline management should be evaluated. Lack of a caregiver or a significant burden on the caregiver they cannot handle is a relative contraindication to implantation. While still poorly understood, frailty is associated with poorer outcomes and it is reasonable to use an objective frailty assessment tool such as the Fried Frailty Phenotype, The Deficit Index, or Handgrip strength test [8]. CT Imaging has been used to measure muscle mass as a surrogate as well [17].

Further, all reversible causes of heart failure should be thoroughly investigated including, but not limited to: treatable coronary disease, arrhythmogenic cardiomyopathy, valvular heart disease, cardiotoxic agents, and infiltrative disorders. The patient's guideline-directed medical therapy should be at maximally tolerated doses and device therapy with cardiac resynchronization therapy (CRT) should be optimized. OHT candidacy should be evaluated. LVAD therapy in advanced heart failure can lead to a significant improvement in quality of life. Follow-up is extensive and complex, requiring a thorough pre-implantation evaluation. Appropriate follow-up requires physicians, nurse practitioners, physical and occupational therapists, as well as social workers [18].

3. LVAD functioning and care

An LVAD is a device that supplants the workload of the left ventricle by pumping blood from the heart to the body. The first generation of LVADs were pulsatile pumps with unidirectional valves that were later transitioned to continuous flow systems due to improved rates of adverse events [19, 20]. Continuous flow LVADs are further divided into axial pumps (propelling blood forward) and centrifugal pumps (moving blood away from pump). Centrifugal-flow LVADs are superior with respect to survival after 2.5 years, gastrointestinal bleeding, and pump thrombosis [21, 22]. The MOMENTUM 3 trial summarized that the newer device system of HeartMate 3 was superior to the previous devices with respect to disabling strokes and the need to replace malfunctioning devices [23].

LVAD implantation requires cardiopulmonary bypass during which the centrifugal pump system is connected to a conduit in the ascending aorta. The pump is connected to an external control unit by a cable called the driveline. The driveline is connected to the pump and tunneled through the abdominal subcutaneous tissue and then to an external controller. The control unit includes batteries and a display of pump parameters [24, 25]. Given the gravity of this intervention, preoperative risk assessment is extensive. It requires optimizations of comorbid conditions and physical fitness. Patients with right ventricular or renal dysfunction may be evaluated in the ICU with invasive hemodynamic monitoring to optimize volume status and end-organ perfusion prior to surgery. The need for renal replacement therapy or mechanical support before LVAD placement is an indicator of higher mortality [11].

4. Post-operative care and monitoring

Immediate post-operative or perioperative care occurs in cardiac or cardiothoracic intensive care units. Optimizing volume status is extremely important in the initial phase as the right ventricle learns to manage the new preload it is exposed to. The LVAD speed is adjusted to optimize the patient's hemodynamics. Typically, the speed is changed with echocardiographic guidance to ensure adequate left ventricular unloading without overloading the right ventricle [25]. The aortic valve should open periodically and minimal mitral regurgitation should be evident.

When titrating the speed, visualization of the interventricular septum is required as the septum should be maintained midline to avoid right ventricular bowing, tricuspid regurgitation, and right ventricular failure. Typical speeds for the HeartMate III are 3000–9000 revolutions per minute (RPM), 6000–15,000 RPM for the HeartMate II, and 2400–3200 RPM for the HeartWare Ventricular Device [26, 27].

Due to mechanisms that are poorly understood, a significant proportion of LVAD patients develop RHF following implantation. Furthermore, RHF plays a pivotal role in the high mortality rates observed among LVAD patients who die from heart failure and multi-organ failure. As a result, in order to optimally manage patients in the post-operative period following surgical LVAD implantation, it is important to understand the pathophysiology of RHF, specifically as it presents in LVAD patients.

Each patient's physiology is monitored on the LVAD monitor via the power, flow, and pulsatility index (PI). Power is the amount of work the LVAD performs to maintain a set speed and typically ranges between 2.5 and 8.5 watts. The flow displayed

Flow	High	High CO	Distributive shock • Infection • Adrenal insufficiency • Vasodilating medications	Volume resuscitation Treat underlying etiology
		Low CO	Aortic insufficiency (AI)	Valve repair
	Low	High CVP	Tamponade Pneumothorax RV failure LV failure • Inflow or outflow obstruction • Pump failure	Treat underlying etiology
		Low CVP	Hypovolemic shock • Hemorrhage • Gastrointestinal losses	• Point-of-care ultrasound for hemothorax, hemoperitoneum, retroperitoneal hemorrhage • Symptomatic control of nausea and vomiting

CO = cardiac output, CVP = central venous pressure.

Table 2.
Unexpected LVAD flows algorithm.

is an estimation with normal values between 2 and 4 L/min. Changes in power and flow outside of the normal range raise concern for pump thrombosis or hypovolemia (**Table 2**). PI represents the strength of left ventricular unloading and is calculated as flow magnitude over 15 seconds with 1–10 being the expected range [25].

Shock in LVAD patients has a slightly different algorithm than in patients without LVADs since the LVAD controller is able to give live time reports. In events where the patient's MAP is less than 60 mmHg, the LVAD flow rate and power should be noted. Simultaneously, cardiac output should be calculated if hemodynamic monitoring is available and bedside echocardiography should be performed [26].

Having a high power with a low flow rate is a strong indicator of possible pump thrombosis. Treatment with thrombolysis, device exchange, or anticoagulation should be considered and implemented immediately. High flow indicator warrants evaluation of cardiac output. In a high flow state with high cardiac output, fluid resuscitation should be started and distributive shock due to infective, vasodilation, or adrenal insufficiency should be considered [26]. If the flow rate is high and the cardiac output is low, then aortic insufficiency (AI) should be evaluated urgently. Decreasing the pump speed would decrease the AI while increasing left ventricular volume. Increasing speed would improve end-organ perfusion while accelerating progression of AI. LVAD outflow cannula diastolic acceleration and systolic-to-diastolic peak velocity ratio correlates well with the true AI severity [28].

The optimal management of cardiac arrest in LVAD patients remains an area of ongoing debate, but a few general principles may be applied in this scenario. Physical exam should be performed promptly to verify the presence or absence of both an audible LVAD 'Hum,' as well as the presence or absence of an arterial pulse by doppler. In the absence of an audible hum or absence of a pulse by doppler examination, ACLS protocol should be

DOI: http://dx.doi.org/10.5772/intechopen.114271

initiated immediately with establishment of an airway by intubation. As chest compressions are a relative contraindication, abdominal compressions have been attempted, but there is limited data to support the efficacy of this method. Postoperative cardiac arrest should be brought back to the operating room without delay [29].

Right ventricular function is thoroughly evaluated prior to LVAD placement (see additional details in 'Patient Selection for LVAD' section above). Postoperative RHF plays a pivotal role in the high mortality rates observed among LVAD patients who die from heart failure and multi-organ failure. As a result, in order to optimally manage patients in the post-operative period following surgical LVAD implantation, it is important to understand the pathology of right heart failure [14].

Favorable hemodynamic changes take place after LVAD implantation, including reductions in left ventricular (LV) and pulmonary artery (PA) pressures. With immediate reduction in LV filling pressures and more long-term remodeling of a long-standing pulmonary hypertension, pulmonary artery resistance goes down, leading to eventual improvement in RV afterload and systolic function. With improved cardiac output, comes increased preload for the RV to accommodate. Chronic right heart failure may result from chronic RV pressure and volume overload. This can occur in the setting of uncontrolled hypertension (excess afterload), excessive LVAD speed, hypervolemia, or any combination of these factors. Tricuspid regurgitation may also be exacerbated by leftward septal shift upon LV decompression which can cause tethering of the tricuspid valve leaflets. RV failure can be precipitated with hypoxemia and increased central venous pressure [14]. This should be evaluated with regular echocardiograms and cautious volume optimization with LVAD speed adjustments, diuresis, or ultrafiltration. Pulmonary hypertension should be treated with phosphodiesterase-5 inhibitors or inhaled nitric oxide [30].

Ramp testing is a formalized protocol that can be utilized to optimize speed and detect device thrombosis. Prior to ramp testing, ensure that the patient is therapeutically anticoagulated with an INR > 1.8 or PTT > 60 seconds. Opening arterial pressure via doppler should be >65 mmHg at baseline. The parasternal long axis view is the primary view used throughout the study. This is due to its optimal position in assessing the LVEDD and LVESD along with the frequency of opening of the aortic valve, any degree of AI or MR, and heart rate. Continuous-flow LVAD parameters are also monitored throughout the study including power, PI, and flow at each stage. Specific speed adjustments for the HMII, and HVAD are given as follows: testing speed range is 8000–12,000 rpm (HMII) and 2200–3200 rpm (HVAD). Start the test by decreasing the speed to 8000 rpm (HMII) and 2300 rpm (HVAD). Give it 2 minutes of washout time, and then evaluate for all the parameters listed above. Perform stepwise increases in speed at intervals of 400 rpm (HMII) and 100 rpm (HVAD) until the upper limit of speed is attained. This will be indicated by LVEDD <3 cm, a suction event or premature ventricular contraction (PVC) beats will occur. PVCs can indicate contact between the LVAD inflow cannula and the interventricular septum (IVS). As stated above, clinically the speed is adjusted to a midline interventricular septum, intermittent opening of the aortic valve as to prevent AI, and minimal MR. Other parameters such as high CVP, low RV stroke work index, elevated pulmonary vascular resistance (PVR), low pulmonary artery pulsatility index (PAPi), high CVP: PCWP ratio, and an elevated diastolic pulmonary gradient have been associated with RHF. The management of RHF can be a multimodal approach to therapy, but generally includes pulmonary artery catheter-guided therapy, aggressive volume optimization using diuretics or even renal replacement therapy when necessary, inotropes, pulmonary vasodilators, heart rate and/or rhythm control, and lastly mechanical RV support in the most severe cases [31].

Options for mechanical RV support include the Impella RP, Protek Duo, peripheral VA ECMO, Paracorporeal CentriMag RV assist device, and durable biventricular assist devices. The timing of when a mechanical RV support device is required varies among centers. One may find that certain centers even preemptively place RV mechanical support in high-risk patients. Others will only offer it once optimal medical therapy has failed. The choice of device also varies depending on the center's practice and experience levels [14].

Anticoagulation in the immediate postoperative period should entail the initiation of intravenous unfractionated heparin within 48 hours of implantation with goal aPTT titrated based on the particular LVAD manufacturer. For example, for the HMII, an aPTT of 40–45 seconds in the first 48 hours, followed by a titration up to an aPTT of 50–60 seconds by 96 hours. For HM III, start heparin 12–24 hours post-implantation with a goal aPTT of 45–50 seconds in the first 24 hours, 50–60 seconds in the subsequent 24 hours, and 55–65 seconds in the subsequent 24 hours. For the Heartware device, begin low-dose heparin at 10 units/kg/h on postoperative day one to target an aPTT of 40–50 seconds and gradually increase to a goal aPTT of 50–60 seconds. Close monitoring of chest tube drainage is key, and a goal aPTT should be adjusted with the quantity of chest drainage in consideration. Heparin is used as a bridge to anticoagulation with Warfarin (vitamin K antagonist therapy). Once a goal INR has been attained with warfarin therapy, heparin can be discontinued. For the HMII, start warfarin within 48 hours of implantation with a goal INR of 2–2.5 by postoperative day 5–7. For the HM III, start warfarin on postoperative day 3–5 once there is no evidence of bleeding and all chest tubes have been removed. A goal INR should be maintained between 2.0–3.0. For the Heartware device, Warfarin should be started within 4 days of implantation with a goal INR 2.0–3.0 [31].

Pump thrombosis is a dire complication and studies have shown increasing fibrous tissues on the LVAD surface due to thrombin generation [32]. As such, anticoagulation is initiated with low-dose heparin and aspirin on post operative day 1 with an aPTT goal 40–60 seconds which is later increased to 60–80 seconds. If no evidence of bleeding, warfarin is initiated after the removal of surgical chest tubes with a goal INR of 2.0–3.0 [33]. Post operative bleeding is an additional complication and management must be cautious as pump thrombosis can have fatal effects. Desmopressin and antifibrinolytics are used, however vitamin K or reversal of anticoagulation should not be considered lightly [34].

Ventricular arrhythmia is another factor that may worsen after LVAD implantation impacting mortality in the first 3 months. It is unclear whether arrhythmias are a sign of hemodynamic compromise rather than the primary cause of mortality [35]. ICD implantation is considered if all other causes of arrhythmias are ruled out and device therapy was not already in place prior to LVAD implantation [36].

Infections in LVAD patients remains one of the most common complications. While a significant proportion of patients developing postoperative infections unrelated to the LVAD had a higher observed mortality, infections of the driveline after 90 days contributes to significant morbidity and affects over 50% of patients at many institutions [37, 38]. In terms of prophylaxis, antibiotic protocols employed in these studies generally favor the use of vancomycin, a cephalosporin, a beta-lactam, and a quinolone. Many centers may also opt for fungal protection as well and add fluconazole. Some centers will even treat MRSA of the nares with mupirocin. Antibiotics prophylaxis is recommended to begin prior to implantation and continue throughout the peri and post operative periods. The major culprits of pocket and driveline infections are gram-positive Staphylococcus species and gram-negative

Pseudomonas species. There were eight retrospective studies and two prospective studies, including one randomized controlled trial (RCT), which describe the optimal antibiotic regimen, however large scale RCTs are needed to assess and validate the efficacy of each regimen [39].

5. Medication management

LVADs contribute to reverse remodeling through various mechanisms. One of those comes from mechanical unloading resulting in improved cardiac output. Simultaneously, the neurohormonal axis begins to normalize with improvement in beta-adrenergic receptor density and reversal of ryanodine-receptor 2 hyperphosphorylation. Additionally, increasing cross-linking of collagen leads to decreased compliance of the left ventricle [40]. This can be augmented with neurohormonal blockade using: angiotensin-converting enzyme inhibitors, B-blockers, angiotensin-II antagonists, neprilisin inhibitors, and aldosterone antagonists. With improved cardiac function, higher doses of these medications can be tolerated to further augment reverse remodeling [41]. Digoxin is also frequently added to this regimen for its ionotropic and antiangiogenesis effects [42].

6. Lifestyle modifications and rehabilitation

Early mobility with physical therapy remains a key to recovery in patients with LVADs. Physical therapy will work with these patients as soon as they are able to participate. Patients work with occupational therapy to ensure that they can perform their self-grooming and may demonstrate the ability to bathe prior to hospital discharge. Rarely, patients may perform well enough to not require discharge to rehabilitation. In patients with a prolonged recovery, cardiac rehabilitation plays a critical role in return to independence. Post-LVAD rehabilitation allows caregivers to continue education in management of this complex device [43].

7. LVAD complications and emergency situations

Strokes, infections, bleeding, right heart failure and device dysfunctions account for most of the long term complications that arise in LVAD patients. Neurologic complications appeared to have the most significant effect on survival with recurring events being detrimental to morbidity and mortality [44]. Patients with high or low INR (>3 or < 1.6), low albumin, or previous stroke seem to be at a much higher risk for post-LVAD strokes. Post-hemorrhagic management is with initiation of aspirin and an individualized approach to determine the safety of further anticoagulation. On the other hand, pump thrombosis leads to embolic stroke, noted mostly in HeartMate II. With the transition to HeartMateIII rates of pump thrombosis have declined [45]. A retrospective study noted the relationship between pre-LVAD cognitive assessment score and 900 day postoperative survival and neurological events [46]. Further evaluation of cognition may be beneficial in improving patient selection and outcomes.

Patients with LVADs are susceptible to postoperative infections, including infections that are unrelated to the LVAD. Infections in patients with LVADs have a significant effect on mortality [47]. After the post-operative course, infection of the driveline is the most dreaded, but almost inevitable complication. Despite attempts at innumerable educational sessions and sterile techniques, driveline infections will frequently occur. Once infected, it is a pathway to LVAD pocket infection as well. The only true treatment for the disastrous development of a device infection is explantation. Patients with controlled infections have been transplanted without a notable increase in mortality risk, but patients rejected due to multidrug resistant infections were not included in this assessment [48]. Most efforts have focused on preventing infection with some benefit to the silicone-to-skin interface at the driveline exit site. Progress in this area is lacking and may partly be due to non-standardized driveline implantation during surgery. Various studies using different antibiotics or horizontal orientation of the driveline have been attempted without significant differences [49].

Gastrointestinal bleeding is a notable comorbidity affecting 24–31% of LVAD recipients. There are no confirmed treatments that reduce its incidence. Some studies noted GDMT to decrease bleeding, however, no association was found during an INTERMACS registry analysis [50]. Acquired von Willebrand Syndrome had a notable increase in the post-LVAD population. Various factors from area of shear stress, to age, CRP, sex, blood type, and time with LVAD did not change prevalence. The effect of this syndrome was investigated in bleeding complications and no association was noted [51]. The typical approach to an LVAD patient with a GI bleed should start with an endoscopy plus colonoscopy, and push enteroscopy if negative. If the source is not found, capsule endoscopy is warranted. In patients with no visible source of bleeding then hemolysis, anemia of chronic disease, or arteriovenous malformations (AVMs) are expected etiologies. In patients with AVMs, antiangiogenic medications can be considered [52].

8. Caregiver support and education

Extensive education is needed before LVAD placement. At times, when the primary implanting LVAD center is not geographically feasible for scheduled follow-ups, a shared care site can be utilized [53]. Caregivers and patients must be educated in anticoagulation management, driveline site inspection and cleaning, and a basic understanding of LVAD alarms. Caregiver support is essential given the high care burden posing a risk for isolation and depression [54].

9. Ethical and palliative care considerations

In patients with heart failure, the end of life is due to failure of the pumping function of the heart. In patients with an LVAD, the end of life is typically due to a complication of their devices. Palliative care providers need to be familiar with these complications to treat their symptoms. Goals of life should be addressed prior to implantation. An LVAD is a heavy burden for the patient and their family and the true cost for all those who will be involved needs to be discussed. Families often need assistance with conversations to determine what their loved one would want once they are no longer able to communicate for themselves and this should be established prior to implantation. It should also be discussed that when choosing comfort care, turning off an LVAD does not equate to assisted death and may or may not lead to an immediate death. It can happen at any location with hospice guidance. Depression in the setting of a high healthcare burden is common and should be monitored and treated [55].

Patients and families without long-term comorbidities have a lower perceived treatment burden [56]. A thorough evaluation of capacity and discussion on all LVAD challenges should occur prior to implantation. While this may not always be possible in emergent situations, the realization of lifestyle changes, recurring hospitalizations, or lack of symptom improvement post-implantation can create an ethical dilemma [57]. Patients have a right to refuse medical care and request LVAD deactivation when that is their desire. Physicians of record should provide resources to respect a patient's wishes in the hospital or at home [58].

10. Future directions in LVAD continuing care

In patients with nonischemic cardiomyopathy, severe HF can be reversed with consideration for LVAD explantation. While recovery is possible at very low rates, relapse rates were high [41].

11. Conclusion

By addressing topics such as LVAD functioning, post-operative care, medication management, lifestyle modifications, complications, caregiver support, and ethical considerations, this chapter aims to provide a comprehensive guide to LVAD continuing care. The information presented will empower healthcare professionals, patients, and caregivers with the knowledge and tools necessary to ensure optimal long-term outcomes for LVAD recipients.

Author details

Michael Sobieraj[1*], Brisha Bhikadiya-Best[2], Sabaa Ahmed[1], Stephen Crawford[1] and Kulpreet Barn[1]

1 Deborah Heart and Lung Center, United States

2 Cooper University Hospital, United States

*Address all correspondence to: sobierajm@deborah.org

References

[1] Chair SY et al. Evolvement of left ventricular assist device: The implications on heart failure management. Journal of Geriatric Cardiology. 2016;**13**(5):425-430. DOI: 10.11909/j.issn.1671-5411.2016.05.015

[2] Severino P et al. Advanced heart failure and end-stage heart failure: Does a difference exist. Diagnostics. 2019;**9**(4):170. DOI: 10.3390/diagnostics9040170

[3] Patel J. Heart failure population health considerations. The American Journal of Managed Care. 2021;**27**(9 Suppl):S191-S195. DOI: 10.37765/ajmc.2021.88673

[4] Aissaoui N et al. Management of end-stage heart failure patients with or without ventricular assist device: An observational comparison of clinical and economic outcomes. European Journal of Cardio-thoracic Surgery: Official Journal of the European Association for Cardio-thoracic Surgery. 2018;**53**(1):170-177. DOI: 10.1093/ejcts/ezx258

[5] Masarone D et al. The ABC of heart transplantation—Part 1: Indication, eligibility, donor selection, and surgical technique. Journal of Clinical Medicine. 2023;**12**(5217):5217. DOI: 10.3390/jcm12165217

[6] Gosev I et al. Long-term survival in patients receiving a continuous-flow left ventricular assist device. The Annals of Thoracic Surgery. 2018;**105**(3):696-701. DOI: 10.1016/j.athoracsur.2017.08.057

[7] Guglin M et al. Evaluation for heart transplantation and LVAD implantation: JACC council perspectives. Journal of the American College of Cardiology. 2020;**75**(12):1471-1487. DOI: 10.1016/j.jacc.2020.01.034

[8] Saeed D, Feldman D, Banayosy AE, et al. The 2023 international society for heart and lung transplantation guidelines for mechanical circulatory support: A 10-year update. The Journal of Heart and Lung Transplantation. 2023;**42**(7):e1-e222

[9] Birks E, Drakos S, Patel S, et al. Prospective multicenter study of myocardial recovery using left ventricular assist devices (RESTAGE-HF [remission from stage D heart failure]) medium-term and primary end point results. Circulation. 2020;**142**:2016-2028

[10] Wasilewski G et al. How to improve the outcomes of LVAD implantation? Transplantation Proceedings. 2022;**54**(4):1054-1057. DOI: 10.1016/j.transproceed.2022.02.052

[11] Liu H et al. Risk stratification and optimization to prevent right heart failure during left ventricular assist device implantation. Journal of Cardiothoracic and Vascular Anesthesia. 2021;**35**(11):3385-3393. DOI: 10.1053/j.jvca.2020.09.130

[12] Cowger JA, Grafton G. Candidate selection for durable mechanical circulatory support. Cardiology Clinics. 2018;**36**(4):487-494. DOI: 10.1016/j.ccl.2018.06.003

[13] Miller M, Crapo R, Hankinson J, et al. General considerations for lung function testing. The European Respiratory Journal. 2005;**26**:153-161

[14] Bravo CA, Navarro AG, Dhaliwal KK, et al. Right heart failure after left ventricular assist device: From mechanisms to treatments. Frontiers in Cardiovascular Medicine. 2022;**9**:1023549

[15] Mendes M. Cardiopulmonary exercise test in the evaluation of heart transplant candidates with atrial fibrillation. Arquivos Brasileiros de Cardiologia. 2020;**114**(2):219-221

[16] Cagliostro M et al. Standardized use of the Stanford integrated psychosocial assessment for transplantation in LVAD patients. Journal of Cardiac Failure. 2019;**25**(9):735-743. DOI: 10.1016/j.cardfail.2019.06.006

[17] Heberton GA, Nassif M, Bierhals A, et al. Usefulness of psoas muscle area determined by computed tomography to predict mortality or prolonged length of hospital stay in patients undergoing left ventricular assist device implantation. The American Journal of Cardiology. 2016;**118**:1363-1367

[18] Hagan K. LVADs: Help mend a broken heart. Nurse Practitioner. 2010;**35**(6):28-37. DOI: 10.1097/01.npr.0000375810.36030.4a

[19] Barić D. Why pulsatility still matters: A review of current knowledge. Croatian Medical Journal. 2014;**55**(6):609-620. DOI: 10.3325/cmj.2014.55.609

[20] Cheng A, Williamitis CA, Slaughter MS. Comparison of continuous-flow and pulsatile-flow left ventricular assist devices: Is there an advantage to pulsatility? Annals of Cardiothoracic Surgery. 2014;**3**(6):573-581. DOI: 10.3978/j.issn.2225-319X.2014.08.24

[21] Masoudi FA. Centrifugal-flow vs. axial-flow LVADs: Two-year outcomes. New England Journal of Medicine. 2018

[22] Goldstein DJ et al. Third annual report from the ISHLT mechanically assisted circulatory support registry: A comparison of centrifugal and axial continuous-flow left ventricular assist devices. Journal of Heart and Lung Transplantation. 2019;**38**(4):352-363. DOI: 10.1016/j.healun.2019.02.004

[23] Mehra MR et al. A fully magnetically levitated left ventricular assist device - final report. New England Journal of Medicine. 2019;**380**(17):1618-1627. DOI: 10.1056/NEJMoa1900486

[24] Singhvi A, Trachtenberg B. Left ventricular assist devices 101: Shared care for general cardiologists and primary care. Journal of Clinical Medicine. 2019;**8**(10):1720. DOI: 10.3390/jcm8101720

[25] Blum FE et al. Postoperative management for patients with durable mechanical circulatory support devices. Seminars in Cardiothoracic and Vascular Anesthesia. 2015;**19**(4):318-330. DOI: 10.1177/1089253214568528

[26] Baronos S, Whitford RC, Adkins K. Postoperative care after left ventricular assist device implantation: Considerations for the cardiac surgical intensivist. Indian Journal of Thoracic and Cardiovascular Surgery. 2023;**39**(Suppl. 1):182-189. DOI: 10.1007/s12055-022-01434-y

[27] Han JJ, Acker MA, Atluri P. Left ventricular assist devices synergistic model between technology and medicine. Circulation. 2018;**138**(24):2841-2851. DOI: 10.1161/CIRCULATIONAHA.118.035566

[28] Grinstein J et al. Accurate quantification methods for aortic insufficiency severity in patients with LVAD: Role of diastolic flow acceleration and systolic-to-diastolic peak velocity ratio of outflow cannula. JACC: Cardiovascular Imaging. 2016;**9**(6):641-651. DOI: 10.1016/j.jcmg.2015.06.020

[29] Garg S et al. In-hospital cardiopulmonary arrests in patients with left ventricular assist devices. Journal of

Cardiac Failure. 2014;**20**(12):899-904. DOI: 10.1016/j.cardfail.2014.10.007

[30] Nair N. Use of machine learning techniques to identify risk factors for RV failure in LVAD patients. Frontiers in Cardiovascular Medicine. 2022;**9**:1-6. DOI: 10.3389/fcvm.2022.848789

[31] Loyaga-Rendon RY, Kazui T, Acharya D. Antiplatelet and anticoagulation strategies for left ventricular assist devices. Annals of Translational Medicine. 2021;**9**(6):521. DOI: 10.21037/atm-20-4849

[32] Spanier T et al. Activation of coagulation and fibrinolytic pathways in patients with left ventricular assist devices. The Journal of Thoracic and Cardiovascular Surgery. 1996;**112**(4):1090-1097. Available from: https://search.ebscohost.com/login.aspx?direct=true&AuthType=sso&db=edsovi&AN=edsovi.00005362.199610000.00028&site=eds-live&scope=site [Accessed: 12 September 2023]

[33] Holman WL, Kociol RD, Pinney S. Postoperative vad management: Operating room to discharge and beyond: In: Mechanical Circulatory Support: A Companion to Braunwald's Heart Disease. Elsevier; 2020:131-143. DOI: 10.1016/B978-0-323-56699-5.00012-7

[34] Muslem R, Leebeek FWG. Bleeding in critical care associated with left ventricular assist devices: Pathophysiology, symptoms, and management. Hematology (United States). 2019;**2019**(1):88-96. DOI: 10.1182/hematology.2019000067

[35] Jedeon Z et al. Association between early ventricular arrhythmias and mortality in destination vs. bridge patients on continuous flow LVAD support. Scientific Reports. 2021;**11**(1):1-8. DOI: 10.1038/s41598-021-98109-2

[36] Allen SJ, Sidebotham D. Postoperative care and complications after ventricular assist device implantation. Best Practice & Research Clinical Anaesthesiology. 2012;**26**(2):231-246. DOI: 10.1016/j.bpa.2012.03.005

[37] Julia BV, Yochiro N, Matthias L. Infections in LVAD patients. Journal of Cardiac Surgery. 2022;**37**(8):2307-2308. DOI: 10.1111/jocs.16591

[38] Choi L et al. Development of an infection-resistant LVAD driveline: A novel approach to the prevention of device-related infections. Journal of Heart and Lung Transplantation. 1999;**18**(11):1103-1110. DOI: 10.1016/S1053-2498(99)00076-5

[39] Acharya MN, Som R, Tsui S. What is the optimum antibiotic prophylaxis in patients undergoing implantation of a left ventricular assist device? Interactive Cardiovascular and Thoracic Surgery. 2012;**14**(2):209-214. DOI: 10.1093/icvts/ivr054. Epub 2011 Nov 30

[40] Pamias-Lopez B, Ibrahim ME, Pitoulis FG. Cardiac mechanics and reverse remodelling under mechanical support from left ventricular assist devices. Frontiers in Cardiovascular Medicine. 2023;**10**:1-12. DOI: 10.3389/fcvm.2023.1212875

[41] Birks EJ et al. Reversal of severe heart failure with a continuous-flow left ventricular assist device and pharmacological therapy: A prospective study. Circulation. 2011;**123**(4):381-390. DOI: 10.1161/CIRCULATIONAHA.109.933960

[42] Abbasi MA et al. Impact of digoxin utilization on clinical outcomes following left ventricular assist device implantation. International Journal of Artificial Organs. 2022;**45**(11):919-926. DOI: 10.1177/03913988221112684

[43] Compostella L, Russo N, Setzu T, et al. A Practical Review for Cardiac Rehabilitation Professionals of Continuous-Flow Left Ventricular Assist Devices: Historical and current perspectives. Journal of Cardiopulmonary Rehabilitation and Prevention. 2015;**35**(5):301-311. DOI: 10.1097/HCR.0000000000000113

[44] Hariri IM et al. Long-term survival on LVAD support: Device complications and end-organ dysfunction limit long-term success. Journal of Heart and Lung Transplantation. 2022;**41**(2):161-170. DOI: 10.1016/j.healun.2021.07.011

[45] Tsiouris A et al. Stroke after implantation of continuous flow left ventricular assist devices. Journal of Cardiac Surgery. 2019;**34**(7):541-548. DOI: 10.1111/jocs.14079

[46] Pavol MA et al. Predicting post-LVAD outcome: Is there a role for cognition? The International Journal of Artificial Organs. 2021;**44**(4):237-242. DOI: 10.1177/0391398820956661

[47] Bini Viotti J, Natori Y, Loebe M. Infections in LVAD patients. Journal of Cardiac Surgery. 2022;**37**(7):2090-2091. DOI: 10.1111/jocs.16576

[48] Copeland H, Baran D. A persistent problem-The dreaded LVAD driveline infection. Journal of Cardiac Surgery. 2022;**37**(1):105-106. DOI: 10.1111/jocs.16075

[49] Shore S et al. Non-patient factors associated with infections in LVAD recipients: A scoping review. Journal of Heart and Lung Transplantation. 2022;**41**(1):1-16. DOI: 10.1016/j.healun.2021.10.006

[50] Jennings DL et al. Impact of heart failure drug therapy on rates of gastrointestinal bleeding in LVAD recipients: An INTERMACS analysis. International Journal of Artificial Organs. 2021;**44**(12):965-971. DOI: 10.1177/03913988211013366

[51] Meyer AL et al. Acquired von Willebrand syndrome in patients with a centrifugal or axial continuous flow left ventricular assist device. JACC: Heart Failure. 2014;**2**(2):141-145. DOI: 10.1016/j.jchf.2013.10.008

[52] Dailey J et al. A multi-center study of left ventricular assist device (LVAD)-related gastrointestinal bleeding. Clinical and Translational Gastroenterology [Preprint]. 2022;**10**:1-7. DOI: 10.14309/ctg.0000000000000526

[53] Yin MY et al. Impact of shared care in remote areas for patients with left ventricular assist devices. JACC: Heart Failure. 2020;**8**(4):302-312. DOI: 10.1016/j.jchf.2020.01.004

[54] Coleman B et al. Vanishing MCS caregiver: Insights into the impact of machines on the caring relationship. Journal of Heart & Lung Transplantation. 2019;**38**:S303. DOI: 10.1016/j.healun.2019.01.761

[55] Warraich HJ et al. Top ten tips palliative care clinicians should know about caring for patients with left ventricular assist devices. Journal of Palliative Medicine. 2019;**22**(4):437-441. DOI: 10.1089/jpm.2019.0044

[56] Warraich HJ et al. Comorbidities and the decision to undergo or forego destination therapy left ventricular assist device implantation: An analysis from the trial of a shared decision support intervention for patients and their caregivers offered destination therapy for end-stage heart failure (DECIDE-LVAD) study. American Heart Journal. 2019;**213**:91-96. DOI: 10.1016/j.ahj.2019.04.008

[57] Guidry-Grimes L, Sederstrom N. Expectation and suffering with LVAD deactivation. The American Journal of Bioethics: AJOB. 2015;**15**(7):74-76. DOI: 10.1080/15265161.2015.1042746

[58] Allen LA. How should physicians respond to requests for LVAD removal? AMA Journal of Ethics. 2019;**21**(5):E394-E400. DOI: 10.1001/amajethics.2019.394

Section 3

Heart Transplantation

Chapter 6

Establishing a Heart Transplantation Program in a Middle East Country: Requirements, Logistics, and Implementation Strategies

Dina Fa Alwaheidi, Tamer Abdalghafoor, Amr Salah Omar, Abdulwahid Almulla, Sankar Balasubramanian and Ali Kindawi

Abstract

Heart failure is a chronic condition that many patients must treat with cutting-edge treatments. Worldwide population growth has increased the demand for various treatments, including heart transplantation. In order to meet the rising demand for such therapy, it was necessary to investigate both local and international options to tackle the increasing rate of HF in the Middle East Region. Local attitudes and perceptions regarding organ donation and transplantation are shifting in tandem with this process. This well-established intervention is not very popular in the Middle East as there are only a few centers that provide this service. We hereby discuss the background and Strategies for heart transplantation requirements, logistics, and implementation in Middle East countries.

Keywords: heart transplantation, regular multidisciplinary review committee, heart donation after brain death, heart donation after circulatory death, ventricular assistant devices

1. Introduction

Heart transplantation has emerged as a lifesaving treatment for end-stage heart failure patients worldwide [1]. Despite the successful outcomes achieved by established heart transplantation programs, many regions, including Middle East countries, lack comprehensive programs for this critical intervention. This chapter will focus on providing an in-depth analysis of the necessary requirements and logistical considerations to establish a heart transplantation program in a Middle East country, with an emphasis on the unique challenges and strategies specific to the region.

Country	First heart transplantation (HT)
Saudi Arabia	The first HT was performed in 1986 at Riyadh Military Hospital [3]
United Arab Emirates	In December 2017, the first successful HT was performed at Cleveland Clinic in Abu Dhabi by a UAE-based team [4]
Iran	Heart transplantation in Iran was first performed in July 1993 [5]
Jordan	In 1985, the first-ever successful cardiac transplant in the Middle East and the Arab world at the King Hussein Medical Center in Amman, Jordan was performed by Dr. Daoud Hanania [6]
Turkey	In 2001, Turkey performed its first successful heart transplant [7].

Table 1.
History of cardiac transplantation in middle east region.

Before we start, it is important to have a vision of the history of heart transplantation in Middle East counties.

Middle East, the lands around the southern and eastern shores of the Mediterranean Sea, encompassing at least the Arabian Peninsula and, by some definitions, Iran, North Africa, and sometimes beyond [2]. According to the published literature regarding the countries providing heart transplant services in Middle East, few countries have this modality of treatment (**Table 1**). In fact, this shows how important it is to work to find new centers and transfer the service to countries that have not yet started the heart transplant program.

2. Infrastructure for heart transplantation program

Building a state-of-the-art facility equipped with advanced cardiac surgery units, dedicated transplant wards, intensive care units, and a comprehensive diagnostic laboratory is crucial [8]. The infrastructure should be designed to meet the unique needs of heart transplantation, including specialized equipment, operating rooms, and dedicated post-transplant care units. Additionally, investing in advanced imaging technologies, such as cardiac MRI and echocardiography, will facilitate accurate pre- and post-transplant assessments.

In addition, complex transplant patients need a large infrastructure that includes specialists in advanced circulatory support, cardiac critical care, nutrition, social work, and other fields. Indeed, a robust, comprehensive, cutting-edge heart transplant program should contain the following components to provide the greatest care for heart transplant patients [9]:

1. Care for all oregonians—modern patient care that is based on public service and does not make distinctions based on insurance status.

2. Adult and pediatric capabilities—able to provide the full continuum of care for patients of all age ranges by being able to address complex heart diseases in both adult and pediatric patients.

3. Multi-organ failure capabilities—access to the knowledge and resources provided on-site by other organ transplantation programs, such as those for the liver, kidney, and pancreas, are crucial for successful outcomes in patients with multiple organ failure.

4. Unmatched expertise—A strong team of advanced heart failure transplant cardiologists, critical care specialists, and transplant surgeons with experience in pre- and post-operative care, who are committed to training future cardiologists and surgeons, need to consistently sharing their knowledge, evaluate current services to ensure best practices, and advance that knowledge.

5. Cardiovascular intensive care unit—around-the-clock intensive care facility that only treats seriously ill cardiovascular patients.

6. Level 1 trauma—patients in urgent need of highly specialized cardiovascular care, including those with heart failure, receive the highest level of round-the-clock lifesaving trauma care.

7. Clinical trials—the capacity to instantly link heart transplant patients with a wide range of clinical trials that offer the most cutting-edge options for therapy in order to support and enhance their care.

3. Legal framework for heart transplantation

Establishing a robust legal framework that addresses organ donation and transplantation is essential. This framework should encompass legislation ensuring the legality, consent, and ethical guidelines for organ procurement and transplantation [10]. It should also include mechanisms for organ allocation and distribution, as well as regulations to prevent organ trafficking. Cooperation with international transplantation organizations and adherence to global standards, such as those provided by the World Health Organization (WHO) [11] and the Declaration of Istanbul [12], is paramount.

For example, in a recent article discussing the legal system in Germany [13] for transplantation, Germany has used the recent organ controversy as a chance to develop its processes for allocating and procuring organs, which are built on the principles of openness, quality assurance, and process improvement. This of course led to Increasing organ donation in Germany, as it depends on winning back the confidence and support of all parties, especially those in the healthcare industry. The German Organ Procurement Organization was strengthened, intensive care specialists were involved in the donation and management of organs, a transplant registry was established, and allocation guidelines were updated, Among the accomplishments to date is a focus on structured specialization training with a future 2-year fellowship requirement, a legal framework for transplant center organization, outcome measures, and quality assurance [8].

4. Medical expertise

Developing a highly skilled multidisciplinary team is critical for the success of a heart transplantation program, multiple professions are engaged in the care of heart transplant patients because of their chronic and complex conditions. This team should include transplant surgeons, cardiologists, anesthesiologists, immunologists, psychiatrists, social workers, and specialized nurses [1]. This is important in the preoperative phase and post-operative care and recovery period. Implementation of

Regular Multidisciplinary Review Committee (MDRC) meetings and daily multidisciplinary rounds for post-operative patients, and expansion of the attendees for the MDRC meetings improved care related to heart transplantation [14]. Collaborations with experienced transplant centers can facilitate training programs, fellowships, and knowledge sharing to build expertise within the local medical community. Establishing partnerships with international institutions for mentorship and guidance can further enhance the knowledge and skills of the transplant team [8].

5. Organ procurement

For decades, the limited availability of heart donors has been an inherent hindrance to cardiac transplantation. As a matter of fact, establishment of a robust cardiac organ procurement system is the most complex task. Hearts procurement is considered a multi-stage process complimented by a series of different interrelated logistics that does not affect donors or recipients only but their families, friends, caregivers, morals, beliefs, and the whole society. Moreover, it's been years before agreeing on science and evidence became clear in setting guidelines to improve the donation numbers. The science of transplantation regarding the safety and availability of donors is evolving, and donors who have not been considered as donors in the past are now able to provide the flair of streaming life to others. Additionally, increasing the number of donors is necessary to increase the number of organs accepted for transplantation by carefully and safely taking into account people who were previously excluded from the process [15].

Current practice entitles two different procurement strategies: the classical strategy; donation after brain death (DBD) and recently; heart donation after circulatory death (DCD) [16].

Donation after brain death (DBD) has been the traditional pathway for years from which hearts have been obtained for transplantation. Unfortunately, most of the reasons resulting in brain death may directly affect the heart, in this regard; a very limited pool of donors has been considered suitable for transplantation. Moreover, the management of this pathway of donation after brain death is complex & it includes keeping cardiac and arterial pressures ensuring a protective ventilation strategy, and homeostasis. People with coronary artery disease (CAD) risk factors, such as age greater than 40, hypertension, a history of using cocaine, heroin, or amphetamines, previous or current smoking history, and dyslipidemia, should undergo coronary angiography; also for patients with a family history of premature CAD; or who have suspected wall motion abnormalities on echocardiography [17]. Each center should advocate a clear criterion to be met to facilitate the procurement decision after reviewing each donor using a specific flow diagram that entitles all information about donor history, all current diagnostic information, and previous and current hemodynamic parameters with continuous repeat assessment of ongoing management, diagnostics & vitals status parameters [18].

On the other hand, heart donation after circulatory death (DCD) is usually perceived as ethically more complex as it necessitates at some point fainting of support from the donor, which might be difficult to explain to the donor's families that a beloved one is kept alive only as a means to convey their hearts to the recipients. Such a concept of keeping and ending life touches on a very sincere tenet in the Middle East society, which values the courtesy of death as much as life. Contradicting misbeliefs and conflicts associated with DCD malefice its implementation in the Middle Eastern world [19].

1. Unfortunately, since organ transplantation was first performed in Egypt in 1976, there has not been a strong legal foundation overseeing it. Organ donation from deceased donors is prohibited by law, so all organ transplant procedures rely on living donors. In addition, a belief that organs cannot be taken from after brain death as life ends with the death of all organs and that as long as the heart still beats, death cannot be declared [20].

   a. In the Kingdom of Saudi Arabia, a person is deemed legally dead under two circumstances: (1) irreversible cessation of cardiac and respiratory function, and (2) irreversible cessation of all cerebral function, as per the Islamic jurisprudence resolution dated October 1986. DCD is therefore not in use in the Kingdom of Saudi Arabia or in the nations of the Gulf Cooperation Council (GCC) [20].

   b. In Kuwait, only DBD has been in practice since the beginning of deceased donor transplantation in 1996.

   c. The Lebanese law No 109/1983 legalizes "donation of human tissues and organs for medical and scientific purposes." DCD has not yet been attempted in Lebanon. Only corneas are retrieved from DCD donors [21, 22].

   d. In Iran, in 1989, it was possible to obtain religious authorization from the Supreme Religious Leader that recognized brain death and permitted deceased-donor organ transplants. Currently, only 1% of donors come from circulatory death [23]. At the Iran University of Medical Sciences, uncontrolled donation after circulatory death (uDCD) was practiced for the first time as of November 2021 [24].

   e. Iraq has been pioneering legislation on organ transplantation and donation in the Middle East. Iraq endorsed a precise legal definition of brain death in 1985; it was improved upon in 1989. Articles describing live and deceased donation, donor criteria, (nonpaid) donation, and consent are included in these laws. However, transplant activities are restricted to live donor transplants that are compatible with their blood group and are still only a live donor program.

   f. According to the Jordanian Ministry of Health law, To be able to perform the necessary procedures, all hospitals with cases of brain death must inform the Jordanian Centre of Organ Transplantation (JCOTD) Directorate [25].

5.1 Beliefs about heart donation

To proselytize such complex belief in a way to show the nobility of gifting life to others stems from convincing people that this transit interim is not by any means agonizing their beloved ones, on the other hand, it might be an interim of salvation and blessing. Building a network that spreads the virtue of charity that lies within the gift of transplantation and the fact that one life can usher hope to many more lives imitated with the religious and ethical principles that might be the obstacle behind the avoidance of transplantation in the Middle Eastern societies. To start with; assessment of awareness and sentiments toward donation should be the first step that would help to prioritize & plan programs and to pass on awareness and spread correct information at community level. Enlighten that those hearts to be harvested immediately after the declaration of death is very important as some people to most of the participants. This will prevent them from wasting precious time to harvest hearts. By incorporating important information and student activities about heart donation within schools and universities, the educational system can be just as important. Religious scholars can be very important because of their significant impact on Middle Eastern society as advocates for heart donation, highlighting misinformation and misperceptions about the position of heart donation in Islam. Targeted campaigns for healthcare professionals, mainly general practitioners, must also be conducted [26].

5.2 Availability of multidisciplinary transplant programs and role of transplant coordinator

Establishing multidisciplinary teams that work regionally & coordinate together is relevant, for example, the transplant coordinator who plays a keystone in the transplant unit & becomes an integral part of its structure through which all relevant information is conducted. Transplant coordinator is often the first person to meet the recipient and to explain the process and might be the last person he sees at the time of clinical discharge. Transplant coordinator should be experienced in the psychiatric and psychosocial assessments, obtaining a psychosocial history, including background, education, work, and current family circumstances is very crucial to begin with & will pave the road while going along this journey [27].

5.3 Health laws framing heart donation

Starting with donation programs that electively include people to list themselves as donors similar to blood donation programs is another way of spreading the idea of transplantation. The willingness to donate heart should be a standard practice in the region similar to some countries that include this information on ID cards rather than giving the choice to next of kin after death. Creating regional networks that function locally and regionally within regions like the Gulf and North Africa to facilitate the availability of heart donation as death due to motor vehicle accidents and cerebral vascular accidents are common and both considered opportunities for cardiac availabilities from brain-dead donors in these areas. In Qatar, A donor registry is been established as a national confidential list of people who are willing to become organ donors after their death [28].

6. Post-transplant care

A small number of centers—one each in Qatar, Egypt, the United Arab Emirates, and two in Saudi Arabia—offer posttransplant care to heart recipients who have received transplants elsewhere and are returning to the region. The Cleveland Clinic in Abu Dhabi, which primarily handles cases requiring transplantation in the United States, currently has the most experience in the Gulf region. Recently in Qatar, they started to develop an integrated post-transplant program that includes cardiologists, surgeons, transplant specialists, social workers, physiotherapists & coordinators who mostly deal with patients who had their transplants in other countries. Gaining experience & learning lessons from such patients who had their transplant outside is crucial to developing the care for those patients who will carry on their transplantation in the region. Fully comprehensive post-transplant care is vital for successful outcomes. Developing a specialized transplant clinics with expertise in immunosuppressive management, infection control, rehabilitation, and long-term follow-up is essential. Collaborations with local healthcare providers and patient support groups can ensure seamless continuity of care. Furthermore, establishing partnerships with international transplant centers can facilitate knowledge transfer and the adoption of best practices in post-transplant care [29].

Post-transplant care is very critical & even more complex than the pre-transplant period. Certain important points need to be framed & stressed:

6.1 Communication and trust

Objective impartial communication channels to be established between patients, their families, and the medical team including a transparent doctor who is compassionate & committed to take the full time needed to alleviate anxiety and build trust from the pre to post-care periods. Centers should offer comprehensive post-transplant care programs. A program that includes support services, education, and counseling to help patients and their families navigate the emotional and physical challenges associated with the transplant process. Full holistic support is critical to address the psychological, emotional, and social aspects of a patient's well-being. These should include support groups, counseling services, and most importantly financial & charity aid to incentivize the willingness to dispute the remodifications encountered during the post-transplant period till recovery. Expertise, hospital reputation, and the patient experience are very crucial in post-transplant care. Tackling all aspects of the potential risks empowers patients to ensure the best possible consequences for such a huge transformative impact on their future lives. Ensuring that post-surgery care does not stop upon discharge but in fact continues at home with check-in appointments, conducting calls with transplant coordinators, and cardiac rehabilitation programs which are all feasible in most of Middle Eastern countries [30].

7. Implementation strategies

A phased approach to program implementation is recommended. Engaging stakeholders early on, conducting feasibility studies, and garnering political and financial support are crucial first steps.

Collaborations with established transplant centers for mentorship and guidance, participation in international conferences and workshops, and leveraging existing resources are effective strategies to accelerate program development [8]. Additionally, establishing partnerships with international organizations, such as the International Society for Heart and Lung Transplantation (ISHLT), can provide valuable guidance and support throughout the implementation process.

This comprehensive overview of the requirements and logistics involved in establishing a heart transplantation program in a Middle East country. It underscores the importance of a multidisciplinary approach, legal frameworks, infrastructure, organ procurement systems, and post-transplant care for successful program implementation. By addressing these key elements, Middle East countries can enhance their healthcare systems, improve patient outcomes, and offer life-saving treatments to individuals suffering from end-stage heart.

8. Ventricular assistant devices

Despite multiple logistic challenges, Ventricular Assistant devices (VADs) as bridge to transplantation have been adopted in many countries across the Middle East region in parallel with other regions in the world. From the real-world data analysis, Heart pumps in Middle East and Africa region are expected to grow with the highest growth rate in the forecast period of 2022 to 2029 due to the upsurge of growing heart awareness campaigns. The heart pump segment in Saudi Arabia is dominating the Middle East and Africa's left ventricular assist device (LVAD) market due to the increasing implantation of mechanical circulatory support devices.

For example, mechanical circulatory support (MCS) program was launched at King Faisal Hospital in Saudi Arabia, 20 years ago. Along with the other two centers that have implanted durable MCS devices as destination therapy, reaching almost a total of 45 durable LVADs per year. Besides, it remains the main heart transplant center in the Middle East, reaching 35 transplants per year with 89% 1-year survival. Other Gulf countries namely Qatar & UAE surged to embrace VADs as treatment strategies as well [31].

In Lebanon, Beirut Cardiac Institute is considered the main local institute that has the widest experience in LVAD in Lebanon, from 2010 to December 2019, 78 patients had different types of VADs, a total of 82 pumps with 4 patients needed an exchange of the pump the reported 12-month survival was 80%, with 75% survival at 18 months, an outcome like the IMACS (International Registry for Mechanically Assisted Circulatory Support) data [32].

Meanwhile, unique challenges complicating the flourishing of such programs also might affect the outcome is the fear of device management at home, on the other hand, in Europe and the US almost every patient is discharged from the hospital awaiting heart transplantation. Also, the burden of other health-related quality of life such as social interaction and Job stability are other important factors that impact decision-making and the future after VADs implantation [33].

9. Conclusions

Heart transplantation services in the Middle East could be improved further if different medical committees in the region worked together to develop a legal framework and share experience and expertise.

Conflict of interest

The author(s) acknowledged no potential conflicts of interest with regard to the research, authorship, and/or publication of this work.

Author details

Dina Fa Alwaheidi[1], Tamer Abdalghafoor[1*], Amr Salah Omar[2], Abdulwahid Almulla[1], Sankar Balasubramanian[1] and Ali Kindawi[1]

1 Department of Cardiothoracic Surgery, Heart Hospital, Hamad Medical Corporation, Doha, Qatar

2 Department of Cardiothoracic Anaesthesia and Intensive Care, Heart Hospital, Doha, Qatar

*Address all correspondence to: tamerabedalghafoor@hotmail.com

References

[1] Ahmed T, Jain A. Heart Transplantation. In: StatPearls [Internet]. Treasure Island (FL): StatPearls Publishing; Jan 2023. Available from: https://www.ncbi.nlm.nih.gov/books/NBK557571/ [Updated 2023 May 22]

[2] Britannica. The Editors of Encyclopaedia. Middle East: Encyclopedia Britannica. 2023. Available from: https://www.britannica.com/place/Middle-East [Accessed: September 25, 2023]

[3] Saudi Center for Organ Transplantation. Organ Transplantation in Saudi Arabia—2015. Saudi Journal of Kidney Diseases and Transplantation. 2016;**27**:1293-1306

[4] Bader F, Atallah B, Rizk J, AlHabeeb W. Heart transplantation in the Middle East Gulf Region. Transplantation. 2018;**102**(7):1023-1026. DOI: 10.1097/TP.0000000000002211

[5] Mandegar M-H et al. Heart transplantation in Iran: A comprehensive single-center review of 15-year performance. Archives of Iranian Medicine. 2009;**12**(2):111-115

[6] Jordanian surgeon transplants heart. Associated Press/Rome News-Tribune. 11 August, 1985. Available from: https://en.wikipedia.org/wiki/Daoud_Hanania

[7] Şahin S, Alkan S. Contribution of Turkey in heart transplant research: A web of science database search. Experimental and Clinical Transplantation: Official Journal of the Middle East Society for Organ Transplantation. 2023;**21**(2):150-157. DOI: 10.6002/ect.2022.0291

[8] Singh SP, Hote MP. Opportunities and challenges for thoracic organ transplantation in government institutions. Indian. The Journal of Thoracic and Cardiovascular Surgery. 2020;**36**(Suppl. 2):210-214. DOI: 10.1007/s12055-019-00808-z

[9] News O. Oregon Health & Science University (OHSU) to reactivate Heart Transplant Program. News, southwest Portland, USA: Oregon Health & Science University (OHSU); 14 Mar 2019. Available from: https://news.ohsu.edu/2019/03/14/ohsu-to-reactivate-heart-transplant-program. In-Text Citation: (News, 2019)

[10] Dew MA et al. The 2018 ISHLT/APM/AST/ICCAC/STSW recommendations for the psychosocial evaluation of adult cardiothoracic transplant candidates and candidates for long-term mechanical circulatory support. The Journal of Heart and Lung Transplantation: The Official Publication of the International Society for Heart Transplantation. 2018;**37**(7):803-823. DOI: 10.1016/j.healun.2018.03.005

[11] World Health Organization. Global observatory on donation and transplantation. Available from: https://www.transplant-observatory.org/ [Accessed: June 10, 2023]

[12] Steering Committee of the Istanbul Summit. Organ trafficking and transplant tourism and commercialism: The declaration of Istanbul. Lancet (London, England). 2008;**372**(9632):5-6. DOI: 10.1016/S0140-6736(08)60967-8

[13] Nashan B, Hugo C, Strassburg CP, Arbogast H, Rahmel A, Lilie H. Transplantation in Germany. Transplantation. 2017;**101**(2):213-218

[14] Roussel MG, Gorham N, Wilson L, Mangi AA. Improving recovery time

following heart transplantation: The role of the multidisciplinary health care team. Journal of Multidisciplinary Healthcare. 2013. pp. 293-302

[15] Hannah Copeland JW, Hayanga A, Neyrinck A, et al. Donor heart and lung procurement: A consensus statement. The Journal of Heart and Lung Transplantation. 2020;**39**(6):501-517

[16] Bernabei A, Tropea I, Faggian G, Onorati F. Donor management and organ procurement. In: Heart Transplantation. Cham: Springer International Publishing; 12 Jan, 2023. pp. 117-128. DOI: 10.1007/978-3-031-17311-0_7

[17] Müderrisoğlu H, Sezgin A. A new concept in donor selection for cardiac transplant patients. Experimental and Clinical Transplantation. 2022;**20** (Suppl. 4):48-50. DOI: 10.6002/ect.DonorSymp.2022.L29

[18] Hobbs RD, Si M-S. Ex vivo heart perfusion for pediatric transplant patients: A new path toward expanding the donor pool for kids? The Annals of Thoracic Surgery. 2021;**112**(4):1281. DOI: 10.1016/j.athoracsur.2021.02.036

[19] Ayer A, Schroder JN, Casalinova S, Doberne JW, Bryner BS, Patel CB, et al. The future of heart procurement with donation after circulatory death: Current practice and opportunities for advancement. The Journal of Heart and Lung Transplantation. 2022;**41**(10):1385-1390. DOI: 10.1016/j.healun.2022.06.016

[20] Haberal M. Donation after circulatory death in Turkey and the Middle East: Current status. Transplantation Reports. 2022;**7**(4):100109. DOI: 10.1016/j.tpr.2022.100109

[21] Jamal AZBHA. Muslim Religious Scholars on the Commodification of Human Body and its Dignity in the Age of Biomedical Revolution (Doctoral dissertation, Hamad Bin Khalifa University (Qatar)); 2019

[22] Kaposztas Z. Donation after circulatory death–activity review in the Asian region. Transplantation Reports. 2022;**7**(4):100122

[23] Ghods AJ. The history of organ donation and transplantation in Iran. Experimental and Clinical Transplantation. 2013;**12**(Suppl. 1):38-41

[24] Malek Hosseini SA. Personal written communication [Accessed: April 5, 2022]

[25] Al Breizat AH. Personal written communication [Accessed: August 10, 2022]

[26] Mekkodathil A, El-Menyar A, Sathian B, Singh R, Al-Thani H. Knowledge and willingness for organ donation in the Middle Eastern region: A meta-analysis. Journal of Religion and Health. 2022;**59**:1810-1823. DOI: 10.1007/s10943-019-00883-x

[27] Afzal Aghaee M, Dehghani M, Sadeghi M, Khaleghi E. Awareness of religious leaders' fatwa and willingness to donate organ. International Journal of Organ Transplantation Medicine. 2015;**6**(4):158-164

[28] Alsaied O, Bener A, Al-Mosalamani Y, Nour B. Knowledge and attitudes of health care professionals toward organ donation and transplantation. Saudi Journal of Kidney Diseases and Transplantation. 2012;**23**(6):1304-1310. DOI: 10.4103/1319-2442.103585

[29] Alkuwari H, Fadhil R, Almaslamani Y, Alansari A, Almaki H, Khalaf H, et al. The Doha donation accord aligned with the declaration of

Istanbul: Implementations to develop deceased organ donation and combat commercialism. Transplantation. 2014;**97**(1):3-4

[30] Qatar Organ Donation Center (QODC). Hiba. Available from: http://organdonation.hamad.qa/en/donation_in_qatar/donation_in_qatar.aspx [Accessed: November 23, 2014]

[31] Sivathasan C, Hayward C, Jansz P, Sibal AK, et al. Durable mechanical circulatory support across the Asia-Pacific region. The Journal of Heart and Lung Transplantation. 2020;**39**(11):1195-1198. DOI: 10.1016/j.healun.2020.08.022. Epub 2020 Sep

[32] Hamdan R, Fakih S, Mohammad M, et al. The Lebanese left ventricular assist device experience, a success story despite the odds. Journal of Cardiothoracic Surgery. 2020;**15**:192

[33] Itzhaki Ben Zadok O, Ben-Avraham B, Jaarsma T, Shaul A, Hammer Y, Barac YD, et al. Health-related quality of life in left ventricular assist device-supported patients. ESC Heart Failure. 2021;**8**(3):2036-2204

Chapter 7

Heart Preservation Techniques for Transplantation

Chawannuch Ruaengsri, Daniel M. Bethencourt, Tiffany Koyano and Yasuhiro Shudo

Abstract

Heart transplant remains the gold standard of end-stage heart failure treatment. The number of heart transplants performed each year has increased and the number of recipient candidates has been increasing even more. As a result, recipients are now matched with donors over longer distances with increasing organ ischemic time. Organ preservation strategies have been evolving to minimize ischemia reperfusion injury following longer ischemic times. This chapter will include updated organ donation and preservation techniques for heart transplant including organ donation after brain death (DBD) and donation after circulatory death (DCD). The expansion of cardiac donation after circulatory death (DCD) and new techniques for heart preservation may increase the use of hearts from extended criteria donors and thus expand the heart donor pool.

Keywords: heart preservation, heart transplant, heart perfusion, heart donation, organ preservation

1. Introduction

The shortage of donors is a major limiting factor in cardiac transplantation [1]. To enlarge the donor pool, extended criteria heart donors, including those with older age, left ventricular hypertrophy, hepatitis B/C infection, donor/recipient size mismatch and prolonged ischemic time are often considered with acceptable outcomes [2]. Organ ischemic time was defined as the time between the aortic cross-clamp applied during procurement and heart reperfusion during heart implantation [3]. Donor hearts are now procured from longer distances; extending the cold ischemic time. The registry of the International Society for Heart and Lung Transplantation report in 2017 demonstrated an ischemic time < 4 hours was associated with improved survival at 30 days and 5 years compared with longer ischemic time [3]. Given older heart donors have been increasingly utilized. Studies have shown that the hearts of older donors are more sensitive to prolonged ischemic time compared to younger donors [4, 5]. Many new strategies have been developed to improve allograft preservation, and minimize the effect of ischemia reperfusion injury. For DCD donors, a period of warm ischemia occurs at the beginning when life support is discontinued. Recently, *ex-vivo* perfusion technology has been developed to minimize warm and cold ischemic times, enable organ resuscitation, evaluation and facilitate long-distance organ transportation. This technology has facilitated the expansion of the donor pool.

2. Heart donation

Heart transplantation was first performed by Christiaan Barnard in 1967 with a DCD approach. The recipient and donor were in adjacent operating rooms. Donor life support was discontinued, and death was pronounced after there was no electrical activity for 5 minutes. The chest was opened, cardiopulmonary bypass was initiated, cardiectomy was performed and the donor heart was perfused through the aortic root until the recipient was ready to implant. The transplant was successful, and the recipient was able to wean off from cardiopulmonary bypass. Unfortunately, the recipient passed away 18 days postoperatively due to pneumonia and acute rejection [6–8].

In 1968, the Harvard Ad Hoc committee included "irreversible coma" to be the criteria for death. Since then, DBD has become the majority method of heart retrieval with the benefit of controlled rapid diastolic cardiac arrest and shorter ischemic time [9]. In 1979, the Stanford team reported the experience of heart procurement at an outside hospital and found it to have equivalent outcomes compared to donor hearts procured in a hospital which led to nationwide organ sharing to increase the donor pool and subsequently decreased waitlist times [10]. The technique of heart preservation after initial cardioplegia infusion was cold storage with topical hypothermia. A Stanford experimental study demonstrated significant ultrastructural changes after 3–4 hours of ischemia which appeared reversible with satisfactory graft function [11].

3. Donor management

The goals of donor management before a heart transplant include maintaining adequate intravenous volume with optimum cardiac filling pressure and ensuring adequate arterial pressure for entire organ perfusion. Arterial and central venous pressure (CVP) lines are essential and should be placed for continuous hemodynamic monitoring and allow blood samples to be obtained as needed. CVP is maintained in the range of 6–10 mmHg to ensure adequate volume status and mean arterial pressure is targeted between 60 and 80 mmHg. All cardiac donors should have an echocardiogram to evaluate cardiac function, LV wall thickness, wall motion and exclude any major structural heart defects. A coronary angiogram is recommended for donors >40 years old or with risk factors for coronary artery disease (smoking, hypertension, hyperlipidemia and methamphetamine users) [12].

Factors contributing to volume depletion include unrecognized blood loss associated with trauma, diminished vascular tone, hyperosmotic therapy from mannitol, third spacing generated by inflammatory mediators, hyperglycemia and diabetes insipidus (DI) resulting in massive diuresis. A total of 0.9% NaCl or Lactated Ringer's solution is generally used in case of fluid depletion. In donors with hypernatremia, 0.45% NaCl or dextrose-containing crystalloids can be used for fluid repletion.

Despite adequate fluid repletion, progressive systemic hypotension still occurs in brain-dead donors requiring vasopressors and inotropes support. Many studies have suggested vasopressin as a first-line drug given simultaneously decreasing DI and catecholamine agonist (V1 and V2) actions [12–14]. Low doses of dopamine may be used as an alternative drug. The study demonstrated the use of dopamine in both kidney and heart transplants was associated with less requirement of postoperative dialysis [15]. Beta agonist treatment should be avoided given the effect of β-receptors down-regulation and subsequently impaired cardiac function post-transplantation [16]. Moreover, hormonal resuscitation (cortisol, anti-diuretic hormone, insulin and thyroid hormone) has been recommended in brain-dead donors [12, 13].

4. Heart dissection and explantation technique

The donor is positioned, prepped and draped from the chin to the pubis. A midline incision is routinely performed for heart and lung dissection procedures along with a midline incision simultaneously made by abdominal surgeon for abdominal organs retrieval. Visual inspection is achieved to evaluate atrial and ventricular sizes, anatomic variations and cardiac contractility. Surface palpation is performed to evaluate coronary artery calcification, ischemic scarring, contusion and to detect thrills or abnormal flows. Pericardial stay sutures are placed bilaterally and secured with snaps on each side to allow lung evaluation in case of concurrent heart and lung retrieval. Some surgeons prefer minimal dissection to avoid arrhythmia and hemodynamic instability that may occur during heart manipulation. Preliminary dissection of key structures is mostly performed on all organs before heparin is given and cannulation. The ascending aorta and the main pulmonary artery are carefully dissected and separated to allow sufficient aortic cross-clamp placement and manipulate the ascending aorta safely and easily. The superior vena cava (SVC) is dissected off the right pulmonary artery circumferentially. The azygous vein is identified and may be encircled, ligated and finally divided after cardioplegia given to avoid massive bleeding. The inferior vena cava (IVC) is dissected to ensure adequate length. All procurement teams should communicate the timing of their preliminary dissection and readiness to proceed to heparinization [17].

Intravenous heparin (400 U/kg) is given before cannulation. The aortic cannulation site is prepared by placing a 4–0 polypropylene purse-string suture. 14 Fr aortic cannular is placed and secured. The antegrade cardioplegia line is de-aired and connected. The SVC is clamped or tied above the azygous vein. The IVC is partially cut. A pool-tip suction tubing should be inserted into the IVC to facilitate abdominal perfusate drainage and prevent right heart distension. To ensure the left ventricle is decompressed, left atrium venting is performed and ensure adequate drainage. If the lungs are not procured, pulmonary veins can be cut at the pericardial reflection. If the heart and lungs are procured in the donor, left atrium venting can be easily performed by cutting the left atrial appendage. To avoid the left atrial appendage cutting, venting of the left atrium can be done by making an incision in the Waterston's groove or left atrial wall, anterior and medial to the left pulmonary veins at the base of the left atrial appendage. When the heart is empty, an aortic cross-clamp is applied. 1–2 L of cardiac preservation solution is delivered at a pressure of 150 mmHg using a pressure bag. The drainage of the left atrium and IVC is checked to ensure adequate perfusion and the left ventricle is decompressed. Inadequate distribution of organ perfusion may cause irreversible allograft damage [17, 18].

If the lungs are procured in the same donor, cardioplegia is given first and the surgeon must ensure the heart is completely stopped before infusing pulmoplegia to prevent pulmoplegic solutions circulating into the coronary circulation. Topical hypothermia is applied in the chest cavity. After infusion is completed, IVC is completely transected then the left atrial incision is made at the Waterston's groove connecting the right inferior and superior pulmonary veins. When the heart is lifted, the next incision is made at the left atrium midway between the lower left and right pulmonary veins confluence and the coronary sinus then extended to the left to the base of the left atrial appendage and connected to the right side. Both heart and lung procurement surgeons must agree before incisions are made to avoid anatomical damages and ensure adequate left atrial cuff for the donor lungs. The SVC is transected proximal to the azygous vein to provide adequate length. The ascending aorta is transected at the aortic arch level. The pulmonary artery is divided at the bifurcation level. The heart is then explanted and transferred to the back table to examine for any surgical damages or anatomical anomalies [12, 17, 18].

4.1 Heart preservation methods

Donor heart preservation is crucial for a successful heart transplantation as measured by graft function and survival [19, 20]. Unlike other solid organs such as liver, kidney or pancreas, cold ischemic time for the heart is limited to 4–6 hours and longer ischemic times adversely affect survival outcomes [21]. Hypothermia slows metabolic rate and cell death by decreasing enzyme degradation which is necessary for cell viability [22].

4.2 Static cold storage

Static cold storage is the most common method of heart preservation worldwide. After the donor heart is visualized and accepted for transplant into the known recipient, careful organ dissection is performed. The ascending aorta is partially dissected off the main pulmonary trunk to be able to apply an aortic cross clamp. The superior vena cava is freely dissected off the right pulmonary artery and the azygous vein is ligated. Intravenous heparin is given before the aortic cross clamp is applied. Cold preservation solution is rapidly delivered through the ascending aorta via a cardioplegic needle to achieve diastolic arrest. Ice slush or cold water is immediately placed for topical hypothermia [17, 20]. The heart is then stored in preservation fluid within sequential sterile bags placed and transported in an ice cooler.

For every 10-degree Celsius temperature reduction, most enzymes of hypothermic animals demonstrate 1.5–2.0 fold reduction in activity according to the Vant Hoff's rule. Still, prolonged ischemic hypothermia decreases the activity of the Na^+/K^+ pump and results in cell swelling. Moreover, cold ischemia stimulates anaerobic glycolysis and glycogenolysis as well as lactic acid production causing tissue acidosis. When tissue perfusion is restored, oxygen free radicals accumulated during anaerobic metabolism contribute to reperfusion cell injury [22]. Several preservation solutions have been developed to minimize these effects with differing electrolytes, supplements and antioxidant concentrations. University of Wisconsin (UW) solution, Celsior solution and Histidine-Tryptophan-Ketoglutarate (HTK) solution are the most common heart preservation solutions utilized in current practice and the posttransplant outcomes among these three solutions have not shown one to be clearly preferable [19, 20].

4.3 Temperature-controlled donor heart transport system

Organ temperature between 0 and 4 degree Celsius maintains high energy phosphates efficiently but there is a significantly increased risk of frostbite or cold injury due to protein denaturation at a temperature below 2 degree Celsius [23, 24]. At higher

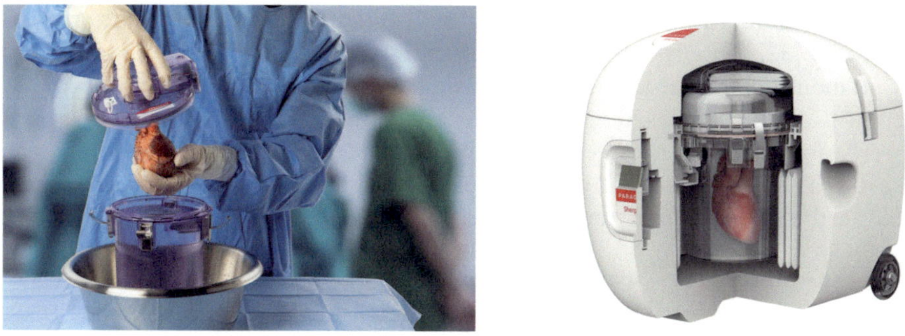

Figure 1.
SherpaPak™ device components. The donor heart is fully submerged in cold preservation solution. Image courtesy of Paragonix technologies, Inc.

temperatures (> 12 degree Celsius), the study showed higher metabolic oxygen demand [24]. To avoid uneven cooling temperature and direct contact with ice, the novel Paragonix SherpaPak cardiac transport system (Paragonix Technologies Inc., MA, USA) was developed and designed to maintain organ temperature from 4 to 8 degree Celsius with special ice packs and temperature sensor. Studies demonstrated that organ storage within this temperature range prevents not only freezing injury and protein denaturization but also decreases metabolic rate and prevents tissue reperfusion injury [2, 23, 25].

The SherpaPak heart transport system (**Figure 1**) is a disposable device and has interchangeable aortic connectors fit for different sizes of hearts. Once the heart is securely attached to the connector, then it is fully submerged in a leak-proof inner canister filled with cold preservation solution. It is then placed in an outer canister surrounded by a specially designed ice pack and protective polystyrene outer shell [26, 27]. The device provides continuous real-time temperature monitoring and transmits temperature and geographic data via Bluetooth connected to a cell phone.

The Stanford team reported the first en-bloc heart-lung transplant using the Paragonix lung guard preservation system, a similar preservation device from Paragonix designed for donor lungs storage. The donor graft was stored in 4 liters of 4 degree Celsius of PhysioSol preservation solution. The average temperature was 7.42 degree Celsius during transport. The recipient was extubated the next day of surgery with good biventricular function and uneventful recovery [28].

After the first clinical study confirmed the safety of SherpaPak used for donor heart preservation with no harmful effect [26], many clinical studies have been conducted to evaluate postoperative outcomes of using SherpaPak for organ transportation [24, 29, 30].

A recent multicentre registry using propensity score matching compared the SherpaPak heart transport system versus traditional static cold storage demonstrated better 1-year survival in the SherpaPak cohort (96.4% with SherpaPak vs. 88.7% with static cold storage). Moreover, significantly fewer patients experienced severe primary graft dysfunction (PGD) requiring an extracorporeal membrane oxygenator (ECMO) in the SherpaPak group resulting in lower overall hospital costs [31].

5. *Ex-vivo* organ perfusion

One of the shortcomings of cold preservation is limited cold ischemic time, with 4 hours generally accepted as safe. The ISHLT database demonstrated that ischemic times beyond 6 hours are associated with graft dysfunction and increased postoperative mortality [32]. *Ex-vivo* heart perfusion was developed based on the Langendorff perfusion model which demonstrated perfusing of coronary arteries was able to resuscitate a dead heart. Based on this concept, a commercial normothermic *Ex-vivo* heart perfusion system (Transmedics Organ Care System, OCS) was developed and recently FDA approved following many clinical trials. Due to its normothermic physiology, the cold ischemic time is lessened while using this platform.

5.1 Normothermic *ex-vivo* heart perfusion

Organ Care System (**Figure 2**) is a portable device with a wireless display monitor. This device consists of a pulsatile pump connected to a gas exchanger and heater which perfuses blood, nutrient solutions and supplements to the organ inside the perfusion module. The PROCEED II was a multicentre randomized trial performed

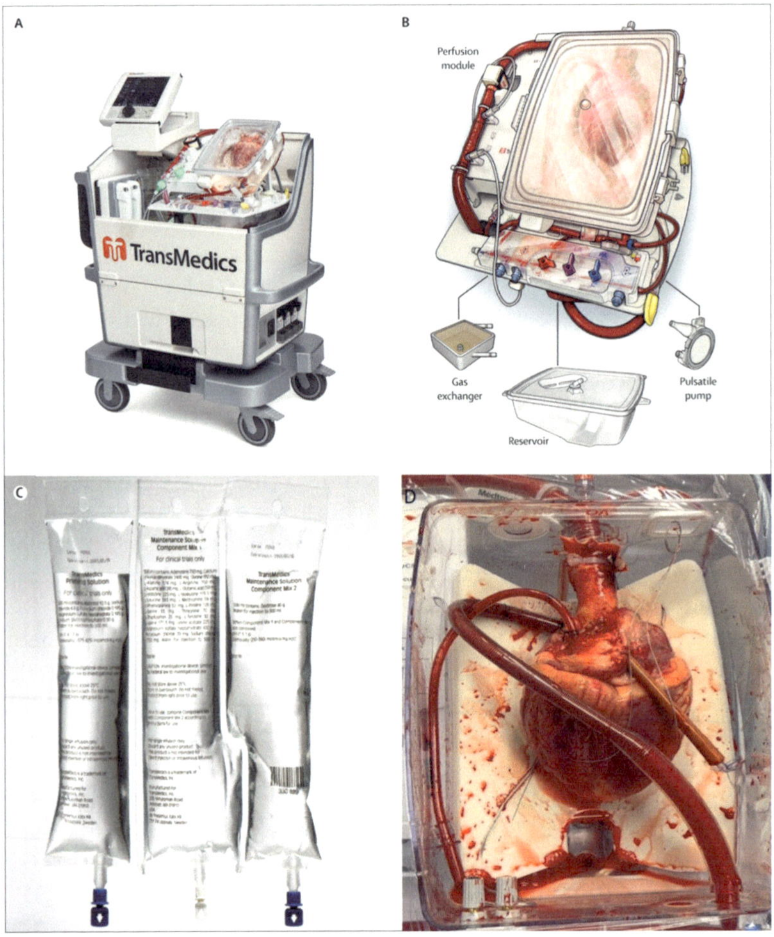

Figure 2.
Normothermic ex-vivo heart preservation, organ care system (OCS) is composed of a portable heart console (A), heart perfusion module (B) and heart solution set (C). The ascending aorta and pulmonary artery are cannulated. The left ventricular vent is placed and secured at the left atrium. The superior vena cava, inferior vena cava, right atrial incision and left atrial appendage are securely closed. The heart is actively beating inside the box (D). This picture has been reproduced by permission of TransMedics (Andover, MA).

in the United States comparing outcomes of the OCS and traditional cold storage, extended criteria donors were excluded. The study showed no significant differences in 30-day mortality, severe graft rejection, ICU stay or cardiac-related complications [33]. At 2 years, the OCS group had a lower survival compared to traditional cold storage but was not statistically different (72.2 vs. 81.6%, $p = 0.38$). There were no significant differences in major serious cardiac events, graft rejection and chronic vasculopathy at 2 years [34].

6. Heart donor recovery

6.1 DBD heart donor using OCS

After a visual assessment for anatomy and function is completed and the heart is accepted for transplant, the aortopulmonary window, superior and inferior vena cava are dissected. Heparin is given and a cardioplegic cannulation is placed. When the donor is ready for aortic cross-clamp, 1200–1400 ml of donor blood is drained into a pre-heparinized blood collection bag for OCS machine priming, using the right atrial cannula with the tip pointed to the inferior vena cava.

After blood collection, the superior vena cava is occluded. The left-sided heart is vented by cutting left the atrial appendage (LAA) or superior/inferior pulmonary vein if the donor's lung is not being recovered for transplant. The right heart is vented from the previous right atrial appendage incision and augmented by cutting the inferior vena cava above the diaphragm. Then, the aortic cross clamp is applied, and cardioplegia is administered through the aortic cannula using a pressure bag to achieve a quick diastolic arrest [17]. Topical hypothermia is applied using ice slush or cold water until cardioplegia is finished. The donor heart is then removed and transferred to the back table for OCS instrumentation [17].

6.2 DCD heart donor using OCS

All necessary surgical instruments and the donor blood collection bag are prepped and set up at the side table before the procedure begins. Heparin 30,000 IU is given 5 minutes before withdrawal of life support. The donor is observed until 5 minutes after electromechanical arrest to ensure a complete cessation of circulation. Median sternotomy is performed quickly, the right atrial cannula is placed in the distended right atrial appendage connected to pre-heparized blood collection bag to retrieve 1200–1400 ml of donor blood using the OCS machine priming.

After blood collection is finished, the aortic cross clamp is applied, cardioplegia is administered, and the right and left heart are vented as described for the DBD donor. Topical ice slush or cold saline is applied. The donor heart explant is performed in a similar fashion as DBD procurement [17]. The donor heart is then transferred to the back table for OCS instrumentation.

6.3 OCS instrumentation

The donor heart is carefully inspected. Patent foramen ovale or any septum defects are carefully checked and repaired if present to ensure the right heart is a closed system for precise coronary blood flow monitoring via pulmonary artery cannula. Any right and/or left atrial appendage incision made previously for blood donor collection and left-sided heart venting are repaired. The superior vena cava is ligated, and the inferior vena cava is then closed using a polypropylene suture secured with a plastic tourniquet. The ascending aorta and pulmonary artery are cannulated. The left ventricle (LV) is vented by placing an LV vent through the left atriotomy.

6.4 Donor heart reanimation and *ex-vivo* preservation

During donor heart instrumentation, the OCS circuit is primed by mixing 1200–1400 ml of donor blood and TransMedics priming solution containing Mannitol and electrolytes. Antibiotics, steroids, albumin and supplements are added to the circuit. Epinephrine, Levothyroxine and the TransMedics maintenance solution containing multivitamins, electrolytes, dextrose, insulin and adenosine are also infused into the system. The aortic cannula is deaired and attached to the circuit with the left atrium and ventricle facing anteriorly. Thirty-four degree-Celsius of oxygenated blood enters and perfuses coronary arteries, returns to coronary sinuses at the right atrium, enters the right ventricle through the tricuspid valve and drains across the pulmonic valve to the pulmonary artery which connected to the pulmonary cannula [35].

After the aortic cannula is attached to the circuit, gentle cardiac massage is usually performed to decompress the heart. At this point, the heart usually starts to beat. If ventricular fibrillation occurs, electrical defibrillation is performed with small defibrillator pads located behind the heart. Biventricular pacing wires are placed, and the ventricular pacing rate is set for VVI at 80 beats per minute. The LV vent is opened and drains into the OCS box connected to the reservoir. When sinus rhythm is achieved, the pulmonary artery cannula is attached to its port [35].

Serial arterial and venous blood gases and lactate are sampled to determine myocardial lactate extraction. A lower venous lactate concentration indicates lactate absorption and reflects adequate myocardial perfusion. Maintenance solution infusion, epinephrine and pump flow are adjusted to keep aortic pressure 65–90 mmHg to maintain coronary flow 650–900 ml/min during transportation. Lactate levels should be absorbing, declining and less than 5 mmol/L before implantation [36, 37].

Once the recipient is ready to implant, the OCS pump is turned off, and cold cardioplegia is delivered to the aortic cannula to achieve rapid electromechanical arrest. The pulmonary artery cannula is disconnected and IVC is opened for drainage to avoid heart distension during the second cardioplegia dosing. After completion of cardioplegia, the aortic cannula is disconnected from the OCS box, and the heart is placed on ice and transferred to the recipient operative field [37].

In March 2023, the Stanford team initiated a new strategy of OCS beating heart transplant without a second cardioplegic arrest to avoid additional ischemic time after heart procurement and to minimize potential ischemic reperfusion injury. This technique can also be applied with DBD heart procurement utilizing OCS. The procedure is performed by perfusing the donor heart with warm blood from the cardiopulmonary bypass circuit via antegrade cardioplegic cannula while the donor heart is still connected to the OCS circuit, then the aortic cross clamp is placed above the antegrade cardioplegia cannula. The donor heart is disconnected from the OCS circuit without interrupting coronary perfusion [36]. The recipient recovered uneventfully with a full return to normal activities at 90 days of follow-up [36].

6.5 XVIVO nonischemic heart preservation device

Rather than perfusing the donor heart beating, with warm solutions using OCS, a Nonischemic Heart Preservation Device (NIHP) is a portable device that perfuses the heart continuously with hypothermic, oxygenated cardioplegia containing blood mixed with a nutrient-hormone solution. XVIVO (**Figure 3**) serves as a mini-cardio-pulmonary bypass circuit consists of an oxygenator, roller pump, heat exchanger, filter and reservoir. The XVIVO consists of the XVIVO Sterile Heart Disposable kit, the XVIVO heart box and the XVIVO supplemented solution. The heart box controls the solution's temperature set at 8° C. The mixed O_2/CO_2 gas flow is supplied to the solution and perfused by the coronary arteries with the control of pressure and flow limits. The sterile disposable kit consists of the tubing, the gas connectors, the pump, pressure and temperature sensors. Machine priming for XVIVO heart preservation system (XVIVO Inc., Gothenburg, Sweden) consists of 2.5 L of supplemented XVIVO heart solution mixed with 500 ml of washed, irradiated leucocyte-depleted red blood cells to achieve a hematocrit of 15%. Heart solution additives consist of sodium bicarbonate, insulin, unfractionated heparin, potassium and imipenem or equivalent broad-spectrum antibiotics. The ascending aorta is cannulated, and connected to the disposable kit then the heart is submerged into a reservoir. The donor heart receives continuous hypothermic oxygenated blood to maintain aortic root pressure at 20 mmHg with 150–250 ml/min of coronary flow in a static, non-beating state [38, 39].

Animal studies have demonstrated the safety of using XVIVO to preserve a porcine heart for 24 hours with at least 8 hours of preserved contractile function and endothelial integrity of the coronary arteries [40–42]. Myocardial contractility and endothelium have been shown to be preserved up to 24 hours with a nonischemic heart preservation device [40].

A nonrandomized phase 2 trial compared six donor hearts perfused with XVIVO and 25 donor hearts perfused with standard cold storage with a median organ preservation time of 223 min in XVIVO and 194 min in the standard cold storage group. The study demonstrated excellent outcomes in XVIVO group with 100% major event-free

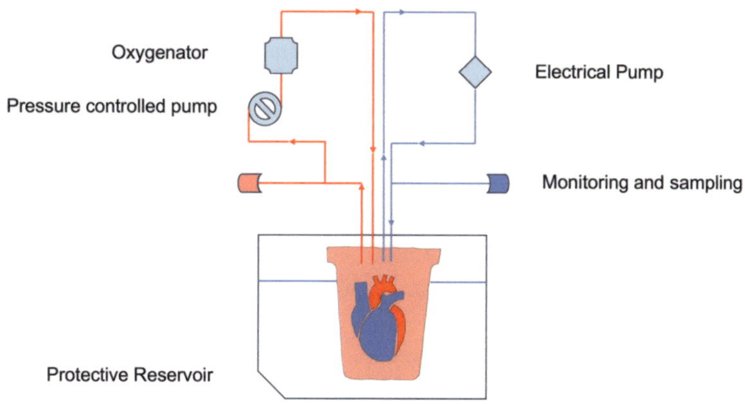

Figure 3.
The XVIVO heart preservation system, the heart is submerged in the cold oxygenated perfusion solution in a protective reservoir. Pressure-controlled pump is used to control the perfusion pressure during perfusion of the heart. The system has integrated sensors that monitor real-time flows, pressures, and temperatures. The picture has been adapted by permission of XVIVO perfusion, Inc.

survival at 6 months (including primary graft dysfunction within 24 hours, need for ECMO within 7 days or acute rejection >2R) compared to 72% major event-free survival in the standard cold storage cohort [38].

XVIVO was used for organ preservation in the first successful pig-to-human transplant by a team at the University of Maryland School of Medicine on January 7, 2022 [43, 44]. Further studies of the XVIVO should be evaluated and compared among the OCS and static cold storage to demonstrate itself as a feasible alternative preservation method. Moreover, this device should be evaluated on extended criteria donors [39].

6.6 Donation after circulatory death (DCD)

Donation after brain death (DBD) has been the primary method of heart procurement. This procedure allows the surgeons to assess visual cardiac function and anatomy and minimizes ischemic injury by controlled cardioplegic arrest. The ISHLT registry data shows that the heart recipient and donor age and comorbidities have been increasing [1]. As demand for heart donors continues to increase, DCD heart donors have become an important alternative in the expansion of the heart donor pool. However, a period of warm ischemic injury occurs during the procurement process when life support is withdrawn to allow electromechanical arrest. DCD procurement techniques and organ preservation methods have been developed to minimize ischemic times [20].

DCD donor categories were classified by the modified Maastricht criteria (**Table 1**) in 1995 [45]. At the present time, DCD donors are classified as controlled DCD or Masstricht category III: Irreversible neurological injury but not meeting the brain death criteria [8, 45–47].

6.7 DCD donation pathway

In most cases, with some variability by hospital policies, 30,000 IU of heparin is administered 5 minutes before withdrawal of life support to ensure it is well circulated (**Figure 4**). Withdrawal of life support can be performed in a post-anesthesia care unit (PACU) or intensive care unit (ICU) to allow participation of family

Category	Sub-category	Definition
Category 1 - Found dead (Uncontrolled)	IA	Unexpected cardiac arrest out of hospital without attempted resuscitation
	IB	Unexpected cardiac arrest in hospital without attempted resuscitation
Category II - Witnessed cardiac arrest (Uncontrolled)	IIA	Unexpected cardiac arrest out of hospital with unsuccessful resuscitation
	IIB	Unexpected cardiac arrest in hospital with unsuccessful resuscitation
Category III - Withdrawal of life support (Controlled)		Expected, planed cardiac arrest after withdrawal of care
Category IV - Cardiac arrest whilst brain dead (Uncontrolled, controlled)		Sudden cardiac arrest following brain death diagnosis but prior to organ recovery

Table 1.
Modified Maastricht criteria for organ donation after cardiac death.

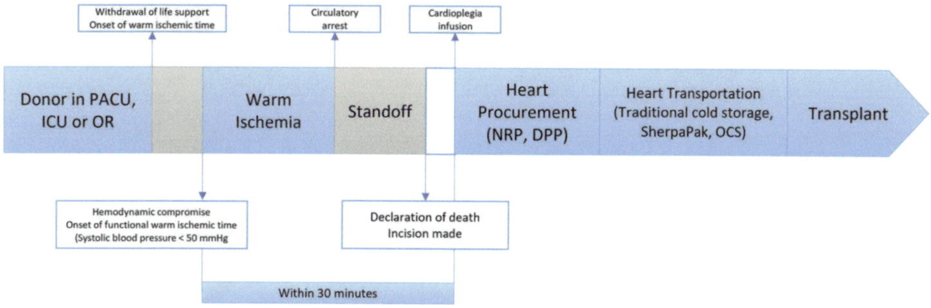

Figure 4.
Donation pathway for DCD.

members depending on hospital policies. In some circumstances, withdrawal of life support is allowed to be performed in the operating theater to minimize warm ischemic time. The donor is then observed for progression of cardiac arrest as indicated by no pulse pressure via an arterial pressure line (mechanical asystole) [8]. The donor is then observed with no interaction (stand-off period) after asystole for an additional 2–5 minutes to ensure the absence of autoresuscitation. Median sternotomy and laparotomy incisions are then performed simultaneously. The warm ischemic time of the DCD donor heart is considered as an end when cold cardioplegia is administered.

Thus "The total warm ischemic time" starts at the time of withdrawal of support and ends when the organ is perfused with cold cardioplegia. "Functional warm ischemic time" refers to the time which the onset of organ hypoperfusion, and typically starts when systolic blood pressure drops below 50 mmHg and ends when cold cardioplegia is infused [45]. Functional warm ischemic time reflects allograft ischemia. Based on previous studies, a DCD heart with functional warm ischemic time exceeding 30 minutes should be excluded from transplant [48, 49].

6.8 DCD reperfusion strategies

A major concern of DCD heart procurement is the potential for myocardial ischemic injury due to prolonged warm ischemic time [45]. Currently, two reperfusion strategies have been utilized to allow functional assessment of donor hearts following circulatory death: Normothermic regional perfusion (NRP) and Direct procurement and perfusion (DPP) using normothermic *ex-vivo* heart perfusion or Organ Care System (OCS) [8, 45, 46].

6.9 Normothermic regional perfusion

This perfusion method likely resembles the first heart transplant technique done by Christiaan Barnard. Once the donor is declared dead, a sternotomy is performed. There are two types of Normothermic regional perfusion (NRP) depending on which organs are planned for recovery. Four units of washed-packed red blood cells are prepared by the hospital blood bank for NRP circuit priming.

1. Thoracoabdominal normothermic regional perfusion (TA-NRP) (**Figure 5**) is used when the heart and/or lungs along with abdominal organs are procured. First, the cerebral circulation is excluded before restoring perfusion by clamping

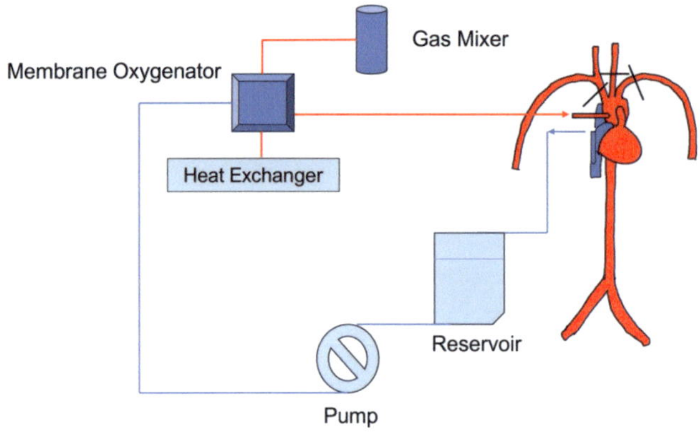

Figure 5.
Thoracoabdominal NRP (TA-NRP). The ascending aorta and right atrium are cannulated. The innominate artery, the left common carotid artery and the left subclavian artery are clamped.

the three cephalic vessels, (the innominate, left common carotid artery and left subclavian arteries). The organs are then re-perfused by initiating veno-arterial extracorporeal membrane oxygenation (VA-ECMO) or cardiopulmonary bypass using central cannulation of ascending aorta and right atrium [48].

2. Abdominal normothermic regional perfusion (A-NRP) (**Figure 6**) is performed if only the abdominal organs are being recovered. The femoral artery and vein or abdominal aorta or inferior vena cava are cannulated. To exclude cerebral perfusion, the abdominal aorta is clamped below the diaphragm. Alternatively, an intraaortic balloon occluder can be used, inserted via the abdominal aorta incision, advanced, and inflated in the thoracic aorta. The inferior vena cava is also clamped to prevent cerebral and thoracic recirculation [50].

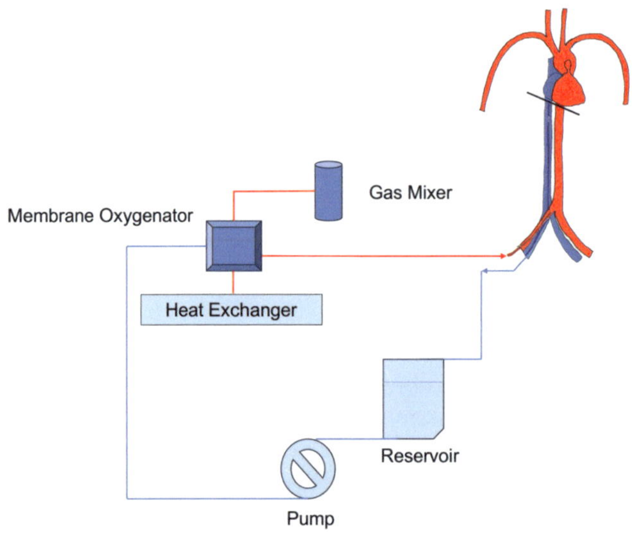

Figure 6.
Abdominal NRP (A-NRP). The femoral artery and femoral vein are cannulated. Veno-arterial ECMO circuit is similar for both Thoracoabdominal NRP and abdominal NRP.

TA-NRP is initiated with the targeted flow at 5 L/min. The heart usually starts beating within 2–3 minutes. If the heart fibrillates, an internal defibrillation (10 J) is delivered. The heart visualization is first inspected. Inotropes or vasopressors are titrated to maintain a mean arterial blood pressure > 50 mmHg. Functional assessment is performed with transesophageal echocardiography (TEE) and pulmonary artery catheter monitoring. The donor is reintubated and ventilated with low tidal volume to avoid atelectasis which would increase pulmonary vascular resistance. As the heart function continues to improve, all inotropes and vasopressors are weaned. Arterial blood gas (ABG) and lactate are obtained to evaluate and confirm adequate perfusion. NRP will continue for 45–90 minutes depending on cardiac contractility [12]. The donor is then weaned off from NRP circuit to visualize unsupported cardiac function. Criteria for acceptance include LVEF ≥50% by TEE, cardiac index (CI) ≥ 2.5 L/min/m^2, central venous pressure ≤ 12 mmHg and pulmonary capillary wedge pressure ≤ 12 mmHg [48]. If the heart is accepted, cold cardioplegia is administered to arrest the heart [51]. Heart explantation and venting are the same as those of DBD heart procurement. For transportation, the heart can be preserved using traditional static cold storage, a temperature-controlled heart transport system or re-perfused with an OCS system [12, 46].

Utilizing OCS after NRP could minimize cold ischemic time compared to using static cold storage. Moreover, in case of complicated redo-sternotomy recipients requiring additional time for mediastinal dissection, OCS provides extra time to achieve a meticulous dissection after the donor heart arrives at the recipient's operating room [50].

NRP provides early continuous physiologic warm blood perfusion, restores cardiac function and establishes perfusion of other organs concomitantly. NRP could reduce the additional cost of *ex-vivo* perfusion machines for each individual organ. Although the NRP is considered less expensive when combined with static cold storage compared with the OCS system [20]. NRP has not been accepted in some regions of the US due to ethical issues related to the NRP protocol (cerebral reperfusion may still occur despite clamping of cephalic vessels [8, 20, 51].

6.10 Normothermic *ex-vivo* heart perfusion

The procurement process and OCS instrumentation are described in the DCD and DBD heart donor technique.

The study of 5-year DCD outcomes showed no differences in 30-day survival (97% for DCD vs. 99% DBD, $p = 1.00$) or 1-year (91% for DCD vs. 89% for DBD, $p = 0.72$). For DCD cohort, there was no differences in MCS use postoperatively (29% in DPP vs. 24% in NRP, $p = 0.75$) but the NRP cohort was found to have shorter ventilator support compared to DPP group (0.5 days in NRP vs. 1.4 days in DPP, $p < 0.01$) [52].

6.11 "Extended criteria" cardiac donors

The demand for heart donors continues to increase but the supply has plateaued [1]. The term "extended heart donor criteria" refers to the expansion of the donor pool by using organs outside of standard categories and using the OCS as a tool to access heart function after explant [48].

The EXPAND trial was conducted to evaluate the safety and efficacy of the Organ Care System in assessing and preserving extended criteria donor hearts [53]. Inclusion criteria include donors with anticipated >4 hours of ischemic time or > 2 hours of ischemic time plus at least one of these following; age > 55 years, 40–50% of ejection fraction (EF), left ventricular hypertrophy, >20 minutes of donor down time. The study demonstrated short-term survival rates were 94.7 and 88% at 30 days and 6 months respectively. The incidence of primary graft dysfunction at 24 hours postoperatively was 10.7% [2, 20, 53, 54].

The limitations of using *ex-vivo* heart perfusion include higher cost compared to the NRP technique and myocardial edema associated with prolonged *ex-vivo* perfusion time, although this effect can be minimized by avoiding unnecessarily high aortic root pressure. Additionally, synchronized pulsatile aortic flow can be used to achieve peak coronary perfusion during the diastolic phase without excessive root pressure [48].

7. Conclusions

Heart transplantation remains the gold standard treatment for end-stage heart failure. Mechanical circulatory support with left ventricular assist devices (LVAD) can provide a bridge to transplantation but has not resulted in the best successful alternative treatment to heart transplantation but adding more risk and complexity during redo-surgery. The demand for heart donors continues to increase and extended criteria donors are being accepted more frequently. Continued research to develop new preservation techniques is crucial to the goals of increasing transport times and expanding the number of donors while preserving optimal allograft function.

Author details

Chawannuch Ruaengsri*, Daniel M. Bethencourt, Tiffany Koyano and Yasuhiro Shudo
Department of Cardiothoracic Surgery, Stanford University School of Medicine, Stanford, CA, USA

*Address all correspondence to: noot@stanford.edu

References

[1] Khush KK, Hsich E, Potena L, Cherikh WS, Chambers DC, Harhay MO, et al. The international thoracic organ transplant registry of the international society for heart and lung transplantation: Thirty-eighth adult heart transplantation report - 2021; focus on recipient characteristics. The Journal of Heart and Lung Transplantation. 2021;**40**(10):1035-1049

[2] Tong CKW, Khush KK. New approaches to donor selection and preparation in heart transplantation. Current Treatment Options in Cardiovascular Medicine. 2021;**23**(5):28

[3] Lund LH, Khush KK, Cherikh WS, Goldfarb S, Kucheryavaya AY, Levvey BJ, et al. The registry of the international society for heart and lung transplantation: Thirty-fourth adult heart transplantation Report-2017; focus theme: Allograft ischemic time. The Journal of Heart and Lung Transplantation. 2017;**36**(10):1037-1046

[4] John MM, Shih W, Estevez D, Martens TP, Bailey LL, Razzouk AJ, et al. Interaction between ischemic time and donor age on adult heart transplant outcomes in the modern era. The Annals of Thoracic Surgery. 2019;**108**(3):744-748

[5] Russo MJ, Chen JM, Sorabella RA, Martens TP, Garrido M, Davies RR, et al. The effect of ischemic time on survival after heart transplantation varies by donor age: An analysis of the united network for organ sharing database. The Journal of Thoracic and Cardiovascular Surgery. 2007;**133**(2):554-559

[6] Buchanan E. The operation: A human cardiac transplant: An interim report of a successful operation performed at Groote Schuur hospital, Cape Town. Author: C N Barnard. South African Medical Journal. 2017;**107**(12):1041-1044

[7] Stolf NAG. History of heart transplantation: A hard and glorious journey. Brazilian Journal of Cardiovascular Surgery. 2017;**32**(5):423-427

[8] Truby LK, Casalinova S, Patel CB, Agarwal R, Holley CL, Mentz RJ, et al. Donation after circulatory death in heart transplantation: History, outcomes, clinical challenges, and opportunities to expand the donor pool. Journal of Cardiac Failure. 2022;**28**(9):1456-1463

[9] A definition of irreversible coma. Report of the ad hoc committee of the Harvard medical school to examine the definition of brain death. Journal of the American Medical Association. 1968;**205**(6):337-340

[10] Watson DC, Reitz BA, Baumgartner WA, Raney AA, Oyer PE, Stinson EB, et al. Distant heart procurement for transplantation. Surgery. 1979;**86**(1):56-59

[11] Billingham ME, Baumgartner WA, Watson DC, Reitz BA, Masek MA, Raney AA, et al. Distant heart procurement for human transplantation. Ultrastructural studies. Circulation. 1980;**62**(2 Pt. 2):I11-I19

[12] Copeland H, Hayanga JWA, Neyrinck A, MacDonald P, Dellgren G, Bertolotti A, et al. Donor heart and lung procurement: A consensus statement. The Journal of Heart and Lung Transplantation. 2020;**39**(6):501-517

[13] Munshi L, Murugan R. Intensive care of the deceased multiorgan donor: One donor, nine lives.

In: Subramaniam K, Sakai T, editors. Anesthesia and Perioperative Care for Organ Transplantation. New York, NY: Springer New York; 2017. pp. 51-61

[14] Plurad DS, Bricker S, Neville A, Bongard F, Putnam B. Arginine vasopressin significantly increases the rate of successful organ procurement in potential donors. American Journal of Surgery. 2012;**204**(6):856-860. discussion 60-1

[15] Schnuelle P, Gottmann U, Hoeger S, Boesebeck D, Lauchart W, Weiss C, et al. Effects of donor pretreatment with dopamine on graft function after kidney transplantation: A randomized controlled trial. Journal of the American Medical Association. 2009;**302**(10):1067-1075

[16] Mascia L, Mastromauro I, Viberti S, Vincenzi M, Zanello M. Management to optimize organ procurement in brain dead donors. Minerva Anestesiologica. 2009;**75**(3):125-133

[17] Shudo Y, Hiesinger W, Oyer PE, Woo YJ. Operative technique and pitfalls in donor heart procurement. Asian Cardiovascular & Thoracic Annals. 2017;**25**(1):80-82

[18] Camp PC Jr. Heart transplantation: Donor operation for heart and lung transplantation. Operative Techniques in Thoracic and Cardiovascular Surgery. 2010;**15**(2):125-137

[19] Li Y, Guo S, Liu G, Yuan Y, Wang W, Zheng Z, et al. Three preservation solutions for cold storage of heart allografts: A systematic review and meta-analysis. Artificial Organs. 2016;**40**(5):489-496

[20] Hess NR, Ziegler LA, Kaczorowski DJ. Heart donation and preservation: Historical perspectives, current technologies, and future directions. Journal of Clinical Medicine. 2022;**11**(19):5762

[21] Minasian SM, Galagudza MM, Dmitriev YV, Karpov AA, Vlasov TD. Preservation of the donor heart: From basic science to clinical studies. Interactive Cardiovascular and Thoracic Surgery. 2015;**20**(4):510-519

[22] Belzer FO, Southard JH. Principles of solid-organ preservation by cold storage. Transplantation. 1988;**45**(4):673-676

[23] Keon WJ, Hendry PJ, Taichman GC, Mainwood GW. Cardiac transplantation: The ideal myocardial temperature for graft transport. The Annals of Thoracic Surgery. 1988;**46**(3):337-341

[24] Michel SG, LaMuraglia Ii GM, Madariaga ML, Anderson LM. Innovative cold storage of donor organs using the Paragonix Sherpa Pak devices. Heart Lung Vessel. 2015;**7**(3):246-255

[25] Ingemansson R, Budrikis A, Bolys R, Sjoberg T, Steen S. Effect of temperature in long-term preservation of vascular endothelial and smooth muscle function. The Annals of Thoracic Surgery. 1996;**61**(5):1413-1417

[26] Radakovic D, Karimli S, Penov K, Schade I, Hamouda K, Bening C, et al. First clinical experience with the novel cold storage SherpaPak system for donor heart transportation. Journal of Thoracic Disease. 2020;**12**(12):7227-7235

[27] Schmiady MO, Graf T, Ouda A, Aser R, Flammer AJ, Vogt PR, et al. An innovative cold storage system for donor heart transportation-lessons learned from the first experience in Switzerland. Journal of Thoracic Disease. 2021;**13**(12):6790-6799

[28] Neto D, Guenthart B, Shudo Y, Currie ME. World's first en bloc

heart-lung transplantation using the paragonix lungguard donor preservation system. Journal of Cardiothoracic Surgery. 2023;**18**(1):131

[29] Bitargil M, Haddad O, Pham SM, Garg N, Jacob S, El-Sayed Ahmed MM, et al. Packing the donor heart: Is SherpaPak cold preservation technique safer compared to ice cold storage. Clinical Transplantation. 2022;**36**(8):e14707

[30] Zhu Y, Shudo Y, He H, Kim JY, Elde S, Williams KM, et al. Outcomes of heart transplantation using a temperature-controlled hypothermic storage system. Transplantation. 2023;**107**(5):1151-1157

[31] Voigt JD, Leacche M, Copeland H, Wolfe SB, Pham SM, Shudo Y, et al. Multicenter registry using propensity score analysis to compare a novel transport/preservation system to traditional means on postoperative hospital outcomes and costs for heart transplant patients. ASAIO Journal. 2023;**69**(4):345-349

[32] Goldsmith KA, Demiris N, Gooi JH, Sharples LD, Jenkins DP, Dhital KK, et al. Life-years gained by reducing donor heart ischemic times. Transplantation. 2009;**87**(2):243-248

[33] Ardehali A, Esmailian F, Deng M, Soltesz E, Hsich E, Naka Y, et al. Ex-vivo perfusion of donor hearts for human heart transplantation (PROCEED II): A prospective, open-label, multicentre, randomised non-inferiority trial. Lancet. 2015;**385**(9987):2577-2584

[34] Chan JL, Kobashigawa JA, Reich HJ, Ramzy D, Thottam MM, Yu Z, et al. Intermediate outcomes with ex-vivo allograft perfusion for heart transplantation. The Journal of Heart and Lung Transplantation. 2017;**36**(3):258-263

[35] Kasinpila P, Ruaengsri C, Koyano T, Shudo Y. Case report: Heart retransplant from a donor after circulatory death and extended transport period with normothermic perfusion. Frontiers in Cardiovascular Medicine. 2023;**10**:1212886

[36] Krishnan A, Kasinpila P, Wang H, Ruaengsri C, Shudo Y, Jackson E, et al. First-in-human beating-heart transplant. JTCVS Tech. 2023;**19**:80-85

[37] Alomari M, Garg P, Yazji JH, Wadiwala IJ, Alamouti-Fard E, Hussain MWA, et al. Is the organ care system (OCS) still the first choice with emerging new strategies for donation after circulatory death (DCD) in heart transplant? Cureus. 2022;**14**(6):e26281

[38] Nilsson J, Jernryd V, Qin G, Paskevicius A, Metzsch C, Sjoberg T, et al. A nonrandomized open-label phase 2 trial of nonischemic heart preservation for human heart transplantation. Nature Communications. 2020;**11**(1):2976

[39] Kothari P. Ex-vivo preservation of heart allografts-an overview of the current state. Journal of Cardiovascular Development and Disease. 2023;**10**(3):105

[40] Qin G, Sjoberg T, Liao Q, Sun X, Steen S. Intact endothelial and contractile function of coronary artery after 8 hours of heart preservation. Scandinavian Cardiovascular Journal. 2016;**50**(5-6):362-366

[41] Steen S, Paskevicius A, Liao Q, Sjoberg T. Safe orthotopic transplantation of hearts harvested 24 hours after brain death and preserved for 24 hours. Scandinavian Cardiovascular Journal. 2016;**50**(3):193-200

[42] Qin G, Wohlfart B, Zuo L, Hu J, Sjoberg T, Steen S. Intact coronary and myocardial functions after 24 hours

of non-ischemic heart preservation. Scandinavian Cardiovascular Journal. 2020;**54**(1):59-65

[43] First successful pig-to-human heart transplant announced. Journal of Clinical Engineering. 2022;**47**(2):65

[44] Wang W, He W, Ruan Y, Geng Q. First pig-to-human heart transplantation. Innovation (Cambridge). 2022;**3**(2): 100223

[45] Ayer A, Schroder JN, Casalinova S, Doberne JW, Bryner BS, Patel CB, et al. The future of heart procurement with donation after circulatory death: Current practice and opportunities for advancement. The Journal of Heart and Lung Transplantation. 2022;**41**(10):1385-1390

[46] Monteagudo Vela M, Garcia Saez D, Simon AR. Current approaches in retrieval and heart preservation. Annals of Cardiothoracic Surgery. 2018;**7**(1):67-74

[47] Shudo Y, Benjamin-Addy R, Koyano TK, Hiesinger W, MacArthur JW, Woo YJ. Donors after circulatory death heart trial. Future Cardiology. 2021;**17**(1):11-17

[48] Beuth J, Falter F, Pinto Ribeiro RV, Badiwala M, Meineri M. New strategies to expand and optimize heart donor pool: Ex vivo heart perfusion and donation after circulatory death: A review of current research and future trends. Anesthesia and Analgesia. 2019;**128**(3):406-413

[49] Colah S, Freed DH, Mundt P, Germscheid S, White P, Ali A, et al. Ex vivo perfusion of the swine heart as a method for pre-transplant assessment. Perfusion. 2012;**27**(5):408-413

[50] Alamouti-Fard E, Garg P, Wadiwala IJ, Yazji JH, Alomari M, Hussain MWA, et al. Normothermic regional perfusion is an emerging cost-effective alternative in donation after circulatory death (DCD) in heart transplantation. Cureus. 2022;**14**(6):e26437

[51] Fiedler AG, DeVries S, Czekajlo C, Smith JW. Normothermic regional perfusion surgical technique for the procurement of cardiac donors after circulatory death. JTCVS Techniques. 2022;**12**:113-115

[52] Messer S, Cernic S, Page A, Berman M, Kaul P, Colah S, et al. A 5-year single-center early experience of heart transplantation from donation after circulatory-determined death donors. The Journal of Heart and Lung Transplantation. 2020;**39**(12):1463-1475

[53] Schroder JN, D'Alessandro D, Esmailian F, Boeve T, Tang P, Liao K, et al. Successful utilization of extended criteria donor (ECD) hearts for transplantation - results of the OCS™ heart EXPAND trial to evaluate the effectiveness and safety of the OCS heart system to preserve and assess ECD hearts for transplantation. The Journal of Heart and Lung Transplantation. 2019;**38**(4):S42

[54] Bryner BS, Schroder JN, Milano CA. Heart transplant advances: Ex vivo organ-preservation systems. JTCVS Open. 2021;**8**:123-127

Chapter 8

Heart Transplantation and Mechanical Circulatory Support in Japan – Past, Current and Future Aspects

Norihide Fukushima

Abstract

The first heart transplantation (HTx) done by Dr. Wada in 1968 misled the general public not to allow to do brain-dead organ transplantation in Japan. It took almost 30 years to issue the Organ Transplantation Act to allow us to perform HTx in Japan. However, this Act required living written consent for brain death and organ donation. Therefore, children younger than 15 years could not donate their organs under brain-dead condition. After 6 years of struggle to revise this Act, the revised Act was issued in 2010 and brain-dead organ donation as well as HTx increased then. But the number in a year has been still extremely less than other developed countries in Japan. Then, we established a special donor management and assessment system to maximize donor organ availability as well as to improve post-transplant outcomes. During these periods, many types of mechanical circulatory supporting (MCS) have been introduced in Japan. Moreover, there have been many developments in immunosuppressive regimens and monitoring to improve outcomes after LVAD implantation and HTx. The chapter will summarize the past, current status, and future aspects of HTx as well as MCS in Japan.

Keywords: heart transplantation, mechanical circulatory support, donor assessment and management, immunosuppressive regimen, organ transplantation network system

1. Introduction

At the beginning of the twenteeth century, when organ transplantation began, the concept of brain death was not widely recognized. Therefore, both the world's first liver transplantation [1] and heart transplantation [2] were performed after cardiac arrest. However, the graft was damaged by ischemia and rejection, and the results were disastrous. On the other hand, the determination of brain death has been discussed since 1957. Then, brain death was proposed as human death, so on June 25, 1968, when the Harvard group announced the definition of brain death, organ transplantation from brain death began in the world.

On August 8 of that year, Japan's first heart transplant was performed at Sapporo Medical University, which caused various controversies. Immediately after the transplant, Professor Juro Wada was hyped up in the mass media for his successful heart transplant. He was started to be accused by the media and public soon after the recipient died 83 days after transplantation. This heart transplant questioned the adequacy of the recipient's indications and the determination of the donor's death. He was indicted in December of the same year but was dismissed after an expert's evaluation was conducted. However, it has caused distrust in transplant medicine based on organ donation after brain death. There were problems with the reaction of the mass media and public opinion, but there were various problems with the Wada heart transplant. It is believed that the fact that these facts were not properly verified has spurred distrust in medical care and has been the reason why organ transplants from brain deaths have become impossible in Japan for many years.

The issues of Dr. Wada's heart transplantation are: (1) whether the recipient was suitable for heart transplantation, (2) whether the donor was truly brain dead, and (3) whether informed consent (IC) had been obtained from the recipient, donor, and their families etc. However, it took more than a decade for the movement to tackle this problem head-on. In 1981, the International Society for Heart Transplantation (ISHT) was established, and in 1982, the Japanese Society for Heart Transplantation was established. Many heart transplants have been performed worldwide, and brain-dead organ transplantation in Japan has come to be actively discussed. In December 1986, the Japan Society for Transplantation published a guideline, "When performing organ transplantation," as a basic provision that should be observed by brain-dead organ transplant recipients in Japan. In October 1987, the Special Committee on Medical Technology and Human Life of the Science Council of Japan announced the "View on Brain Death". In January 1988, the final report of the Japan Medical Association's Bioethics Roundtable was presented and approved by the board of directors, but there were objections from some doctors, and the medical community did not reach a consensus. In 1989, the Japanese Society of Thoracic Surgery established a special committee on organ transplantation to examine problems and solutions in Wada's heart transplantation and published the 1st edition of "Heart and Lung Transplantation - Summary Report on Technical Evaluation and Bioethics" (1991) and the second edition (1992).

As a result of these discussions, it was found that under the current system in Japan, regarding the issue of Wada's heart transplantation (1), to register brain-dead organ transplant patients, the approval of the central indication review committee is required, and strict determination of recipient eligibility is required. This is done so that patients who are not eligible for organ transplantation do not undergo transplant surgery. As for (2), the most stringent legal standards for determining brain death in the world have been established, and brain death is determined by specialists who are neither attending physicians nor transplant doctors. As for (3), IC for recipients and families is maintained at each facility, and IC for donor families belongs to the Japan Organ Transplantation Network, which is independent of donor facilities and transplant facilities, or has received a transplant. The donor coordinator is doing it.

2. Enactment and revision of the "organ transplantation act" in Japan

Since its establishment in 1985, the Legislative Council for Bioethics Research has been researching this issue. In March 1988, when it had reached an extremely important social stage, the Liberal Democratic Party's Policy Research Committee launched the "Research Committee on Brain Death, Bioethics, and Organ Transplant Issues," based on the belief that it was important for the legislature to deliberate comprehensively and carefully. In 1990, the Ad Hoc Brain Death and Organ Transplant Research Committee was established within the Prime Minister's Office. In January 1992, a report entitled "Important Matters Concerning Brain Death and Organ Transplantation" was submitted, stating that brain death should be medically, socially, and legally defined as human death. Said, "It is not something that cannot be implemented without a law, but it is desirable to develop legislation such as the Organ Transplant Act (provisional name)." It has been submitted. When this law was enacted, the House of Councilors made amendments such as "Brain death is considered human death only in the case of organ donation," and "It is necessary for the person to indicate in writing their intention to accept the determination of brain death." In June 1997, the Organ Transplantation Act was passed.

During this period, the Joint Committee of Transplantation-Related Academic Societies was established to certify transplant facilities and to consider recipients, donor eligibility criteria, and recipient selection criteria. Furthermore, it is necessary to conduct a two-stage review because it is necessary to strictly select recipients, and in addition to the hospital review of transplant applicants, a committee has been set up in the Japanese Circulation Society to review indications for heart transplantation, and it is essential to determine the indications there. The Joint Committee of Transplantation-Related Academic Societies approved the Osaka University-National Cerebral and Cardiovascular Center joint team and Tokyo Women's Medical University as initial heart transplant facilities.

The Organ Transplant Act was enforced on October 16, 2009. At the same time, the Japan Kidney Transplantation Network was reorganized as the Japan Organ Transplantation Network, and registration of applicants for heart, liver, and lung transplants began. Under this organ transplantation law, the donor needed to express his/her intention to donate in writing. In addition, according to civil law, the age at which a will can be made is valid for people aged 15 and over, and people under the age of 15 cannot donate, and heart transplants for younger children cannot be performed.

The first heart transplantation [3] based on the Organ Transplant Act was performed at Osaka University on February 28, 1999, and the second [4] was performed at the National Cerebral and Cardiovascular Center on May 12, 1999. Since then, the number of cases has gradually increased from a few to more than 10 per year, but in 2003, not a single heart transplant was performed. On the other hand, the number of people who wanted a transplant was increasing, and the waiting period had been getting longer. Many adults as well as children went abroad and had a heart transplant in the U.S.A and Germany.

At that time, a movement to revise the law began to be seen in the Diet in 2003, led by Diet member Taro Kono, who had donated his liver to his father. On February 25, 2004, the Bioethics and Organ Transplantation Committee approved that "if the patient's intention is unknown, brain-dead organ donation is possible with the consent of the family." On the other hand, in addition to the Japan Society for Transplantation, various academic societies that are responsible for patients with severe organ failure established the Council of Organ Transplantation-Related Academic Societies as a community in November 2003, and patient groups are also actively involved in organ transplantation. Activities for revision have been started. As a member of the Future Planning Committee of the Japanese Society for Transplantation, the author of this chapter was going to make petitions to Diet members one by one with members of patients' organizations related to transplantation. We created pamphlets and videos for petitions and distributed them to councilors of transplant-related academic societies.

In March 2005, the investigative committee stated three items as the skeleton of the revised Organ Transplantation Act, such as (1) organ donation is possible with the consent of family members regardless of age if the individual did not express a refusal to donate before death, and (2) if a donation will be expressed in writing before death, he/she can preferentially donate organs to his/her spouse or relatives within the second degree of kinship, and (3) an organ donation column on driver's licenses and insurance cards will be set up. It was decided that the discussion would be entrusted to the "Organ Transplant Study Group" consisting of volunteers from the Liberal Democratic Party and New Komeito. From March to April of the same year, hearings were held with experts from various fields. At that time, there was an opinion that the chairman of the Japan Pediatric Society Yoshikatsu Eto, and the Japanese Nursing Association had not agreed to regard brain death as human death. On April 28 of the same year, "if he/she has not indicated a refusal to donate, he/she can donate organs with the consent of his/her family regardless of age." was added (commonly known as Plan A) [5].

Although the details after that were omitted in the chapter, every country in the world has a shortage of organ donors, and the pros and cons of traveling overseas for transplantation have become a problem. In May 2010, the World Health Organization issued a new guideline on organ transplantation, putting pressure on legislation. However, what moved the members of the Diet the most was the fact that the parents of three boys who died while preparing to receive heart transplants abroad or after they had traveled abroad went to the Diet, saying, "Parents who lose their beloved children no more." I do not want you to make it."

As a result, the Revised Organ Transplant ACT was enacted in July 2009 and enforced in July 2010. With this revision, it is now possible to donate organs with the family's consent if the person's intention is unknown, and it is now possible to donate organs from children under the age of 15 who have been determined to be brain dead. In addition, as a criterion for selecting recipients, if an organ donation is received from a person under the age of 18, priority will be given to applicants who have registered under the age of 18 for heart transplantation. In February 2014, the recommended age for heart transplantation was raised from under 60 to under 65.

3. Development of mechanical circulatory support for advanced heart failure in Japan

Artificial heart development research was carried out in 1957 by Akutsu and Kolff at the Cleveland Clinic [6], and ventricular assist device (VAD) was carried out by Kusserow [7].

Atsumi et al. of the University of Tokyo started research and development of an extracorporeal pulsatile VAD in Japan at about the same time and in 1980 it was clinically applied at Mitsui Memorial Hospital. Subsequently, Takano et al. of the National Cerebral and Cardiovascular Center (NCVC) also developed the other extracorporeal pulsatile Nipro VAD (Nipro Co. Ltd., Osaka, Japan) and it was clinically applied at NCVC in 1982 [8]. Both VADs began clinical trials in 1986 as bridges to recovery (BTR) for acute heart failure or cardiogenic shock, and both were covered by insurance in 1990. In 1992, when this VAD was applied to a 16-year-old boy with dilated cardiomyopathy, VAD for the purpose of a bridge to a heart transplant (BTT) was not covered by insurance. The patient later traveled to the United States and underwent a heart transplant, who is still alive today. A pulsatile flow implantable VAD, the Novacor (World Heart Corp., Oakland, CA) was the first to be reimbursed for BTT purposes in Japan (2004). It took a long time to get approval after the clinical trial, and it was no longer produced in the United States. In 2006, we withdrew from the Japanese market. However, it must not be forgotten that the fact that the implantable VAD was reimbursed by insurance at this time the home management fee was approved, and although the amount was small, the medical fee of this implantable VAD implantation was approved. It was the cornerstone of the current implantable VAD treatment. Moreover, the first heart transplantation under the Japanese Organ Transplant Act was performed on a 47-year-old man supported by a Novacor VAD for more than 4 months [3]. Meanwhile, another implantable VAD, the HeartMate XVE (Thoratec Corp., Pleasanton, CA) has completed clinical trials but has not been reimbursed. Following the reimbursement of this implantable VAD, the Nipro VAD has also been approved for use for BTT purposes.

Around this time, the mainstream changed from pulsatile flow VAD to non-pulsatile flow VAD in Europe and the United States. and was launched in 2008 and was reimbursed in April 2011 in Japan. As a result, the mainstream of VAD in Japan has become non-pulsatile flow implantable VAD [9]. After that, Jarvik 2000(Jarvik Heart, Inc.; New York, NY), HeartMate-II (Thoratec Corp., Pleasanton, CA), and HVAD (HeartWare Inc., Framingham, MA) were reimbursed one after another. As a result, it can be said that implantable VAD treatment can be performed according to the patient's physique, pathology, etc. After introducing the HeartMate 3 (Thoratec Corp.; Pleasanton, CA) for BTT use, HeartMate 3 became the most popularly used VAD for BTT purposes as well as destination therapy (DT) purposes which were reimbursed by insurance in April 2021.

For children, Nipro VAD, HVAD, or Jarvik 2000 can be fitted depending on their physique. Reimbursed, but currently out of production). In April 2015, Berlin Heart EXCOR VAD (Berlin Heart, The Woodland, TX) was reimbursed by insurance, which can be implanted in infants. The implementation of the revised Organ Transplant Act in 2010 made it possible to donate brain-dead organs from children under 15 years of age [5]. Then infantile heart transplantation has started since 2012 and 27 children supported with EXCOR LVAD and one with Biventricular ECOR VAD had transplantation at the end of 2022.

4. Social and medical system of heart transplant medicine

4.1 Heart transplant facility

Heart transplantation facilities are deliberated by the Council of Heart Transplant/ Cardiopulmonary Simultaneous Transplantation Associations, which consists of the Japanese Circulation Society, etc., and the facilities deemed appropriate as heart transplantation facilities are recommended by the Joint Committee of Transplantation Associations and certified. be.

As of the end of 2022, there are 11 certified facilities. Five can perform transplants for all ages: the National Cerebral and Cardiovascular Center, Osaka University, the

University of Tokyo, Tokyo Women's Medical University, and Kyushu University. The other 5 can perform transplants for patients 11 years old and over, Hokkaido University, Tohoku University, Chiba University, Nagoya University, and Saitama Medical University International Medical Center. The last one can perform transplants for children who are listed under the age of 11: National Center for Child Health and Development There are a total of 11 facilities.

4.2 Indications for heart transplantation and registration with the Japan organ transplantation network

With the introduction of β-blockers and ACE inhibitors, the prognosis of severe heart failure has remarkably improved, and the eligibility criteria for heart transplantation have been reexamined. In Japan, the system is such that a patient is registered in the Japan Organ Transplantation Network after it has been approved through a two-step review by the transplant institution's adaptation review committee and the Japanese Circulation Society Heart Transplantation Adaptation Review Subcommittee.

4.2.1 Indications for heart transplantation

Severe heart disease that cannot be expected to save or prolong life with conventional treatment methods such as dilated cardiomyopathy (DCM), dilated phase hypertrophic cardiomyopathy (dHCM), ischemic myocardial disease, restrictive cardiomyopathy, secondary cardiomyopathy (post myocarditis, drug-induced and postpartum), and congenital heart disease that cannot be surgically repaired, etc.

The indicated diseases in Europe and the U.S.A are divided into cardiomyopathy and ischemic heart disease, which is different from cardiomyopathy accounting for more than 90% of registered cases in Japan. According to various statistics, the number of patients eligible for heart transplantation in Japan is estimated to be 228-670 per year, and the prognosis of these patients is poor, with a 1-year survival rate of around 50%.

4.2.2 Eligible conditions for heart transplantation

Eligible conditions include (a) heart failure requiring long-term or repeated hospitalization for incurable terminal conditions; (b) NYHA grade III-IV heart failure that does not improve with conventional therapy including beta-blockers and ACE inhibitors; (c) patients with fatal severe arrhythmia who are ineffective against any existing treatment. The patient should be under the age of 60 at listing.

4.2.3 Exclusion criteria for heart transplantation

(a) Severe disease other than the heart (hepatorenal dysfunction, chronic obstructive pulmonary disease, malignant tumor, severe autoimmune disease, etc.), (b) Active peptic ulcer or infection, severe diabetes, severe obesity, and severe osteoporosis (c) alcoholism, drug addiction, neuropsychiatric disease, and (d) severe pulmonary hypertension (recent pulmonary infarction, severe irreversible pulmonary vascular disease, etc., drug (prostaglandin, nitroprusside)), a pulmonary vascular resistance coefficient of 6 units or more, or a transpulmonary artery pressure gradient of 15 mmHg or more, even if oxygen or nitric oxide is used) are not indicated.

5. Organ transplant network

a. *Role of the Japan Organ Transplant Network (JOT)*

Regarding brain-dead organ donation, a network system that distributes them fairly and equitably is necessary. In response to this, it plays the role of an organ placement agency. More than 30 donor coordinators belong to JOT, and one to several prefectural organ transplant coordinators are appointed in each prefecture to handle donor information from organ donation facilities and identify donor candidates. Explain heart donation to the family and obtain consent for heart donation. Other tasks include updating the registration of transplant applicants, searching for recipients, following up on transplant recipients, establishing hospital systems at organ donation facilities, and raising awareness among the general public.

b. *Renewal of registration for transplant applicants*

Transplant applicants are registered after evaluating the suitability of each organ, but in particular, for the heart, the transplant facility applies for transplant request registration to JOT after the suitability study of the Japanese Circulation Society's transplant suitability review system. In other words, registration is done when the receipt of the transplant applicant registration form and the payment of the transplant applicant registration fee of 30,000 yen are confirmed.

Also, after registration, renewal procedures are required once a year. In other words, once the transplant request registration renewal form has been received and the payment of the renewal fee of 5000 yen has been confirmed, it will be renewed, and you will be a candidate for the next year. If it is not renewed for 2 consecutive years, it will be canceled. In addition, there is a system of exemption from registration fees and renewal fees for households on public assistance or households exempt from residence tax by submitting the prescribed documents.

c. *Selection of recipient*

Recipients are selected according to recipient selection criteria for each organ stipulated by the Ministry of Health, Labor, and Welfare. Heart transplant recipient selection criteria were established when the Organ Transplantation Act was enacted in October 1997, and after several revisions, were finally revised in November 2012.

First, as matching conditions, ABO blood group identity (identical) and compatibility (compatible) are targeted, and matching is given priority over matching. In addition, a weight difference (donor/recipient) of −20 to +30% is desirable, but the actual selection does not exclude cases outside that range and is a case-by-case decision. In adults, transplantation from a 20% smaller female to a larger male has been identified as a risk factor for premature graft failure. On the other hand, in the case of children, even if there is a large weight difference, the decision is made on a case-by-case basis. If the donor's heart is large, the number of days until chest closure and the length of stay in the ICU tends to increase, but it is said that there is no effect on the survival rate.

In addition, a lymphocyte direct cross-match test (direct cross-match) is carried out at the transplant testing center using the donor's T-cell lymphocytes and the recipient's T-cell lymphocytes, which are blood-collected and cryopreserved in advance. The recipients whose test is positive are excluded from the recipient list. In addition, if there is a blood transfusion within the last 4 weeks, it is necessary to conduct a new direct lymphocyte crossover test using fresh blood. If the panel test (PRA) test is negative, the lymphocyte direct crossover test can be omitted, but currently, all cases are not omitted and the lymphocyte direct crossover test is performed.

Since it is desirable that the permissible ischemic time is within 4 hours, transportation means will be arranged with a goal of 2 to 3 hours for transportation from the donor facility to the transplant facility.

The recipient's medical urgency is divided into three, Status 1 is the state of wearing a ventricular assist device, an intra-aortic balloon pumping, and extracorporeal membrane oxygenation, the state of being under mechanical ventilation management, or the state of requirement of intensive care receiving continuous administration of inotropic drugs in the intensive care unit. For registrants under the age of 18, even if they are receiving continuous administration of inotropic drugs but are not in the critical care unit, they will be registered as Status 1 (however, if they reach the age of 18 in this condition, they will be registered as Status 2). Status 3 is a state in which the registrant of Status 1 or 2 is temporarily removed from the list due to an exclusion condition such as an infectious disease. Status 3 returns to the original Status when the exclusion condition is resolved. Regarding age, heart donations from donors under the age of 18 will be given priority over applicants under the age of 18 at the time of enrollment. In addition, heart donations from donors aged 18 and over are given priority to applicants under the age of 60 at the time of registration. If medical urgency, age, and blood type are the same, the order of the list of Status 1 registrants is defined by the Status 1 waiting period and that of Status 2 registrants is defined by the total number of days from the date of registration.

6. Donor evaluation and management to maximizing heart availability

6.1 Medical consultant system

Among brain-dead donors, only 20% meet the standard donor criteria for all medical conditions. Therefore, to solve the shortage of donors, it is important to make it possible to transplant marginal donor organs. In other words, the purpose of donor management is not simply to stabilize the hemodynamics of the donor until the surgical resection, but to enable the donation of as many organs as possible, improve the organ function of the marginal organs, and improve the organ function after transplantation. This allows many transplant recipients to benefit from organ transplantation. At the same time, it fulfills the wishes of donors and their families, who want to donate as many organs as possible. However, if the recipient dies early after the transplant by forcing the transplant, the donor family feels that they have lost their family once again. Do not forget that the donor family will feel guilty if the recipient dies soon after transplantation. In other words, eliminating primary graft failure (PGF) is important not only for the recipient but also for the donor and their family.

In Japan, since November 2002, medical consultants (MCs) have introduced the system [10] and have been conducting meticulous evaluation and management of donors. After the first determination of brain death, the MCs are dispatched to the donor hospital, evaluate the donor, and manage the donor from the second determination of brain death. Since the basics of donor management are respiratory and circulatory management, donor management is performed by heart and lung transplant doctors, but organ evaluation may be requested by the MC of each organ as necessary. At the beginning of 2002, the number of MCs was small, but now JOT entrusts MCs to 2 persons from each heart transplant facility, 3 persons from each lung transplant facility, and several transplant doctors for other organ transplants.

After obtaining the consent of the donor family to donate brain-dead organs, the MCs received the first call before the first brain-death determination began and arrived at the donor hospital. If the donor's hemodynamics are unstable, JOT coordinators consult with the MCs to stabilize it, and if requested by the donor hospital, MCs attend an apnea test and support hemodynamics management.

6.2 Donor management

6.2.1 Management of hemodynamics

There is no drug therapy that restores the organ viability and function in a short period of time, and it is extremely difficult to restore function after the organ has been removed. Improving organ function and restoring organ function are the mainstays of donor management. Again, why the hemodynamic/respiratory condition is poor should be evaluated first, and the treatment should be determined based on the evaluation results. Drugs that increase peripheral vascular resistance, especially noradrenaline, reduce blood flow in abdominal organs and worsen perfusion of organ preservation solutions, so the dose should be reduced as much as possible. Preservation of cardiac function is achieved by adjusting preload and afterload, administering anti-diuretic hormone (ADH) (details described later), and keeping the dose of catecholamine at the minimum maintenance dose (DOA 10 μg/Kg/min or less as much as possible).

The target values for hemodynamics are (1) systolic blood pressure of 90 mmHg or more, (2) central venous pressure (CVP) of 6–10 mmHg, and (3) hourly urine output of 100 ml/hr. (or 0.5–3 ml/kg/hr).) above, (4) Heart rate 80-120 beats/minute.

6.2.2 ADH replacement therapy

When the ADH blood concentration decreases, (1) diabetes insipidus, (2) a decrease in vascular tone, and (3) a decrease in the affinity of myocardial β-adrenergic receptors, resulting in unstable hemodynamics. Although there are reports that ADH is supplemented only in patients with diabetes insipidus, ADH should be administered even in cases of low urine volume in order to improve (2) and (3). Similar to the administration of ADH after open-heart surgery or in shock during sepsis, the administration of ADH improves hemodynamics, which in turn improves renal function, which often results in an increase in urine output.

Regards to the administration method of ADH, there are reports that it is administered to the bolus by intranasal administration or intramuscular injection, hemodynamics are well stabilized by initial intravenous administration of 0.02 U/Kg (or 1 U) as a bolus followed by continuous intravenous administration (0.01-0.2 U/Kg/hr. or 0.5-1 U/hr). If hemodynamics is stabilized after administration of ADH while maintaining systemic blood pressure of 90 mmHg or more and urine output of approximately 1-2 ml/Kg.hr., r catecholamines are tapered in the order of noradrenaline and adrenaline. As endogenous and exogenous adrenaline levels decrease, the heart rate stabilizes at around 90-120 beats/minute. If the urine output drops sharply after starting ADH, the dose of ADH is reduced. There are many reports of discontinuing ADH before surgical resection, but discontinuation of ADH may lead to a sudden increase in urine output or decreased adrenaline sensitivity in the myocardium and blood vessels, resulting in intraoperative hemodynamic instability. Therefore, ADH administration is discontinued just before heparinization.

6.2.3 Respiratory management

Acute lung injury (ALI) and adult respiratory distress syndrome (ARDS) occur due to the occurrence of various systemic inflammatory reactions before and after brain death, and the sympathetic nervous system is overexcited (sympathetic/autonomic storm) in 15. -20% of brain-dead persons. In addition, due to the denervation, atelectasis easily develops, and pneumonia is likely to occur unless endotracheal suction is carefully performed. In addition, diabetes insipidus can lead to pulmonary edema when excessive hydration leads to a decrease in serum oncotic pressure.

Ventilator settings were made to maintain partial pressure of arterial oxygen (PaO2) of 100 mmHg or more by setting a low fraction of inspiratory oxygen (FiO2) and positive end-expiratory pressure (PEEP) of 5 cmH_2O or to maintain PaO2 of 70-100 mmHg or more, SaO2 of 95% or more, PaCO2 at 30-35 mmHg and pH of 7.35-7.45 by setting tidal volume of 10-12 ml/Kg and maximum airway pressure of 30 mmHg or less. Keeping oxygen concentration, tidal volume, and PEEP as low as possible reduces the inflammatory response in the lung and is thought to improve lung function after transplantation.

Because airway neural reflexes (cough reflex, etc.) are lost, regular repositioning and airway suctioning are important in preventing pulmonary infections and atelectasis. Atelectasis is especially likely to occur in the back of the body. However, in brain death, the cardiac and vascular reflexes are lost, so postural changes and endotracheal suctioning (fluctuations in airway pressure and blood return to the lungs) can easily cause blood pressure to fluctuate, making airway management difficult. Hemodynamic instability is even more difficult to manage, so replenishing ADH and stabilizing hemodynamics are also important in terms of respiratory management.

If the cough reflex is lost, deep sputum aspiration becomes insufficient, so bronchoscopic tracheal/endobronchial aspiration is important. Taking regular chest X-rays (generally every 6-8 hours), observing the progress of atelectasis and pneumonia, and repeating endotracheal aspiration not only improves the condition of the transplanted lung but also reduces the size of the lung. Increased availability.

6.2.4 Correction of electrolytes, hematocrit, and blood sugar

It is well known that hypernatremia adversely affects liver and pancreatic function. In the heart, Hoefer et al. [11] reported that the 1-year survival rate of heart transplant recipients from donors with Na $<$ 130 mEq/l and $\geq$ 170 mEq/l was significantly lower than those from donors within the normal range. and normalizing Na is important. Na-free (or low-Na) transfusion is often performed to correct hypernatremia, but this alone is not sufficient, and it is important to achieve natriuresis by correcting ADH. Correct the serum Na level to a target of 135-150 mEq/l.

When diabetes insipidus occurs and the circulating blood volume decreases, a large amount of transfusion is required, the blood is diluted, and hypokalemia and anemia are likely to occur. First, while treating diabetes insipidus with ADH, it is important to periodically measure the serum K level and replenish K through the central route. Correct the serum K value to about 3.8-4.5 mEq/l. If short-term correction is unavoidable, it may be necessary to administer KCl in a double dilution (0.2 mEq/kg/hr) with a syringe, but this should be administered with careful monitoring. Generally, as diabetes insipidus improves, the serum K value often normalizes. Since anemia impairs organ function, blood transfusion should be performed so that the hematocrit is 30% or higher.

When brain death occurs, the adrenaline concentration in the blood increases, and various inflammatory reactions occur, making it easy to develop hyperglycemia. Suspect hyperglycemia if urine output does not optimize even after correcting ADH. Treatment is first with non-glucose transfusions, and if the condition is still not optimized, continuous intravenous administration of insulin (regular insulin 0.5-1.0 IU/hr). Blood glucose is corrected to target 120-180 mg/dl.

6.2.5 Body temperature control

When brain death occurs, body temperature cannot be regulated, so it is easy to fall into hypothermia. This is particularly noticeable after hypothermia of the brain or when a large amount of fluid is infused due to diabetes insipidus. Compensate for 35.5-36.5°C.

6.2.6 Control of infectious diseases

Long-term brain death can easily lead to pneumonia from atelectasis and infections from bedsores and various catheters. Therefore, in addition to endotracheal suctioning, postural changes to prevent bedsores and care for various catheters, wounds, and bedsores are important. If infection is suspected, ask for bacteriological examination (preferably culture) and administer sensitive antibiotics. Cultivation takes time, so smear examination (a Gram stain is sufficient) is helpful. Antibiotics are started 1 hour before leaving the ward to increase blood levels of antibiotics immediately before skin incision for excisional surgery.

As a result of such careful donor evaluation and management, the average number of organs donated from one donor is 5, which is more than in Europe and the United States (average of 3_4 organs). It seems that the wish of the donor family is also fulfilled.

7. Heart procurement surgery

Although it is a system unique to Japan, after each organ procurement team has completed the evaluation of the transplanted organ at the intensive care unit of the donor hospital, the donor hospital administrator/attending physician, operating department nurse, anesthesiologist (respiratory and cardiological management doctor), each organ procurement team, JOT Cos, et al. have gathered together to hold a meeting on organ procurement surgery. After self-introduction, the procedure for procurement of each organ, line of resection (pulmonary artery and vein, aorta, and superior and inferior vena cava), drainage method, dosage and timing of drugs (antibiotics, heparin, and steroid), organ transport method and scheduled hospital departure time are confirmed. As a result, a very smooth procurement operation is performed. As a result of this meeting, the procurement surgery start time is determined, which in turn determines the recipient's surgery start time. At the same time, we are reaffirming our respect for the donor and her family. A cardiologist assists with cardiorespiratory management during the surgical excision.

In Europe and the United States, surgeons perform surgery in the order of arrival at the donor hospital, but in that case, the heart extraction is often started later, which sometimes makes the donor's hemodynamics unstable and results in giving up heart extraction. In Japan, all procurement teams perform surgery together after arrival. When the surgery start time is decided, consent for organ donation is obtained from the donor's family again, and the donor is transported to the operating room. At this time, it is customary for the entire procurement team to greet the donor and his/her family at the entrance of the operation department to show the utmost respect to the donor and his/her family. After a JOT Co finally confirms that the donor's family has agreed to the donation, all members observe a moment of silence before starting the operation. After all the organs have been removed, the chest and abdomen are closed in the clinically usual way, and the operation is discontinued after a moment of silence. Doctors accustomed to organ donation in Europe and the United States may think that it is not necessary to go that far, but the author thinks that it will continue as a custom that was born from the unique culture of Japan that respects the "heart". As the author mentioned to Co in the U.S.A., Southern California recently observed a moment of silence at the beginning of an operation. When transporting the heart, a cooler box is used to ensure that the heart functions better, and the cooler box is wrapped in a cloth and transported as if it was the donor's remains. This might be not enough to convey our gratitude to the donors and their families who donated their hearts, but we hope to convey our gratitude. Sometimes, for families who want to say goodbye to their hearts in the box for the last time, we arrange a moment of farewell to their hearts just before the heart board an emergency vehicle or helicopter. Because the heart has a short safe tolerance time, it is often airlifted by helicopter or airplane, arriving at the transplant hospital within 3 hours, within 4 hours the donor's heart is beating again, and within 1 hour the heart pulsation becomes stronger and the recipient can be weaned from the heart-lung machine. At that point, in most cases, the donor's family is still staying at the donor hospital, so the recipient Co at the transplant hospital will inform the JOT of the withdrawal from cardiopulmonary bypass so that the information will be available to the donor family. After knowing that the loved one's heart was beating strong in the recipient's body and knowing that the recipient's family was grateful, the donor family made their way home. We believe that it will reduce the grief of the family.

8. Care of heart transplant recipients

In principle, a heart transplant is a brain-dead organ donation, and it is a necessary condition for the recipient to cherish the heart that has been received. Although it depends on the progress after the transplant, the recipient should not forget to convey his/her gratitude to the donor's family with a thank-you letter. In order to take good care of the heart that has been given to the recipient, it is essential to take care of complicated oral treatment, various periodic examinations (including myocardial biopsy), meticulous self-management (consideration of diet and infectious diseases), and smoking cessation. By being grateful to the donor/donor family, the recipient will be able to thoroughly manage his/herself, and as a result, the recipient will be able to live a long and healthy life.

Young children often do not decide to have a transplant by themselves and are prone to non-compliance and anxiety during puberty, so it is important to provide support that matches their mental development. Transplant patients are susceptible to infectious diseases, so it is important to take preventative measures against infectious diseases. However, if infectious diseases become prevalent at schools, they will be forced to take long-term absences from school, so cooperation with schools is important. As appropriate, we meet with staff at the educational institution (including school nurses, nurses, etc.) to ensure that the child is not excluded from class. The fact that the recipient takes good care of the heart that was given to them and, as a result, lives a long and healthy life, is a great way to show gratitude to the donor and the family, and to be happy for the donor's family as well.

9. Outcome of heart transplantation

9.1 Outline

In February 1999, the first heart transplant was performed by the Organ Transplant Act, but the number of organ donations was small, remaining at around 10 per year. In July 2010, the Revised Organ Transplantation Act was enacted, and with the increase in the number of brain-dead organ donations (**Figure 1**), the number of heart transplants increased, reaching 84 in 2019, and decreased to 54 cases in 2020 and 59 cases in 2021 (**Figure 2**). On the other hand, since April 2011, a

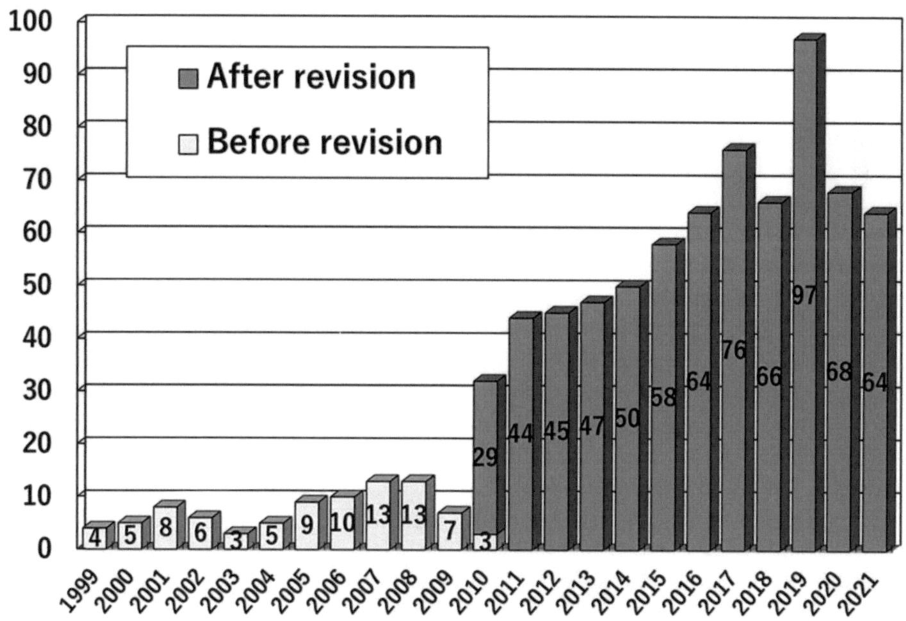

Figure 1.
Brain-dead organ donation performed in Japan by year (up to December 31, 2021) before and after implementation of the revised organ transplant act.

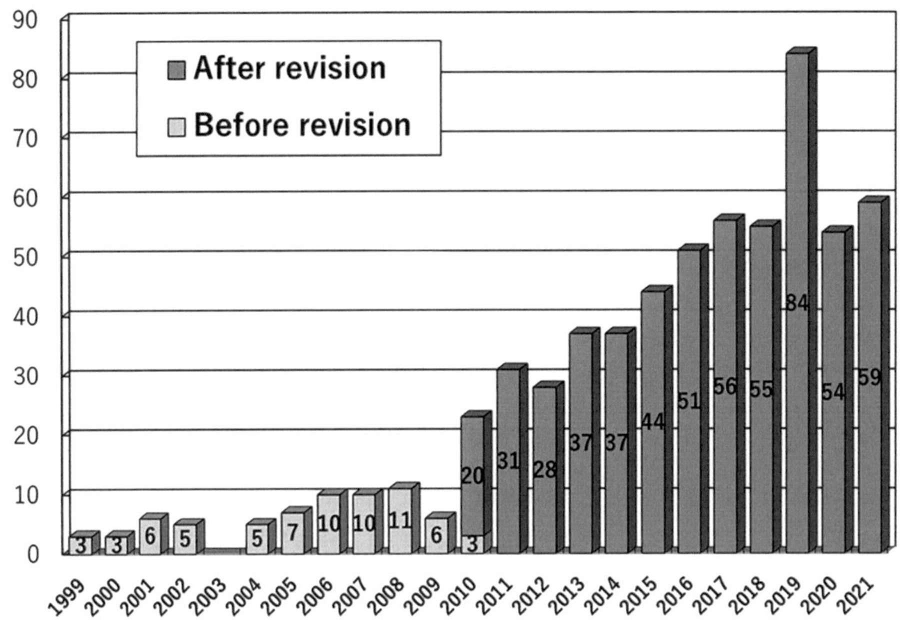

Figure 2.
Heart transplantation performed in Japan by year (up to December 31, 2021) before and after implementation of the revised organ transplant act.

relatively small non-pulsatile implantable VAD that can be treated at home has been reimbursed by insurance as a BTT. Since the increase in the number greatly exceeds the number of transplants, the waiting period for transplantation is increasing. At the end of August 2022, excluding 3 children after the enforcement of the revised Organ Transplantation Act, the cases are limited to Status 1 cases with high medical urgency, regardless of whether they are children or adults. Heart transplant request registration to the JOT began in October 1997, and by the end of June 2022, 2218 cases had been registered, of which 659 had undergone heart transplantation, 71 had undergone overseas transplantation, and 50 had undergone overseas transplantation. 517 cases have died, with cases being deregistered due to worsening conditions.

With the implementation of the revised law, it became possible to donate brain-dead organs from children under the age of 15, and heart transplants from children under the age of 6 began to be performed in 2012 and Berlin Heart EXCOR was reimbursed in 2015. As pediatric brain death organ donations gradually increased, 17 pediatric heart transplants were performed in 2019 and the number of pediatric cases (under 18 years old) reached 60 in total at the end of 2021 (**Figure 3**). The waiting period for transplantation was also shorter than that for adults.

9.2 Changes in the number of heart transplants

9.2.1 Enforcement case

The first heart transplantation based on the Organ Transplant Law was performed in February 1999 [3], and 3 cases were performed in the same year [4]. Since then, the number of heart transplants has increased from around 5 to around 10 per year,

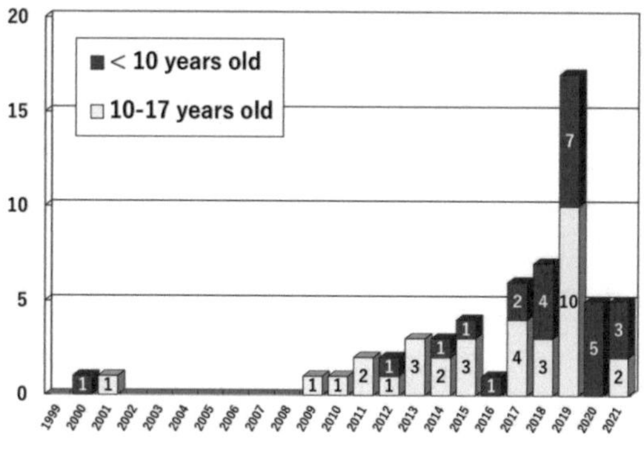

Figure 3.
Pediatric heart transplantation performed in Japan by year (up to December 31, 2021) (by recipient age).

and the amended Organ Transplant Act was enacted in July 2010, resulting in a marked increase in organ donations from brain-deceased patients [9], and 84 heart transplants in 2019. Of these, 17 children were performed, but the number decreased to 59 due to the impact of the new coronavirus infection (**Figure 2**). By December 31, 2021, 625 heart transplants had been performed, including 446 males (71%) and 179 females (29%), with ages ranging from 1 to 70 years (average 39.1). there were. <10 years: 26 cases, 10-19 years: 48 cases, 20-29 years: 88 cases, 30-39 years: 118 cases, 40-49 years: 160 cases, 50-59 years: 133 cases, 60-69 years Age: 51 cases, age 70 or older: 1 case. Currently, patients under 65 years of age are registered for heart transplantation, but due to the long waiting period, there were 4 patients aged 65 years or older (the oldest was 70 years old) who were transplanted.

9.2.2 Medical condition during waiting heart transplantation

Most of the heart transplant cases in Japan are BTT cases, and initially, the Nipro VAD was mainly used. After introducing implantable non-pulsatile VAD in 2011, non-pulsatile flow implantable VADs that can be treated at home, such as HeartMate 3, HVAD, EVAHEART, and Jarvik 2000, are mainly used. Therefore, of the 625 cases at the time of heart transplantation, only 3 were children with status 2, 35 were on inotropic agents, and 587 (94%) were BTT cases (including 46 children). BTT cases now account for 71% (444 cases). On the other hand, the number of pediatric cases transplanted from EXCOR Pediatric gradually increased to 6 cases in 2019 and 3 cases in 2021. The survival rate after installation of a non-pulsatile flow implantable VAD is high (3-year survival rate of 87%), and the number of waiting patients is increasing year by year. Of the 56 patients who underwent heart transplantation in 2015, 18 had been supported with a VAD for 4 to <5 years, 21 for 5 to <6 years, and 8 for 6 years or longer prior to heart transplantation (**Figure 4**).

9.2.3 Cardioplegia and transplant surgery

Modified Collins solution, St. Thomas solution, Bredshneider solution, UW solution, and Celsior solution have been used as cardioplegic solutions, but since 2006, Celsior solution has been used at all facilities other than Kyushu University. Lower-Shamway method, bicaval method, modified-bicaval method, etc. are used as surgical methods. The modified-bicaval method, which was developed in Japan [12], has been used, including in pediatric cases, except where the method is being used.

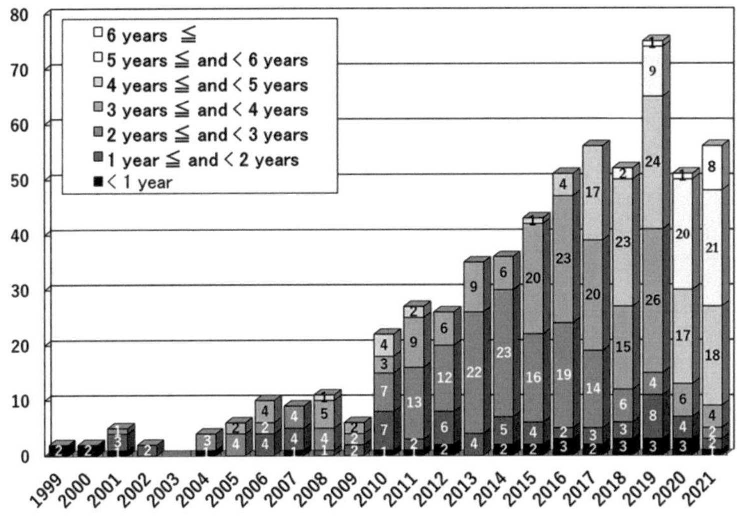

Figure 4.
Heart transplantation in patients supported with left ventricular assist device (LVAD) performed in Japan by year (up to December 31, 2021) (by support year of LVAD).

9.2.4 Immunosuppressive regimen

For induction therapy (including children), anti-CD3 antibody (monoclonal anti-CD3 antibody: OKT3), anti-lymphocyte globulin (ALG), and basiliximab have been used. Although 230 of 625 cases (37%) have been treated with basiliximab, insurance coverage as induction therapy for renal dysfunction cases and pediatric cases described later is awaited.

Initial immunosuppressive therapy was a triple therapy using a calcineurin inhibitor (CNI), cyclosporin (CyA) or tacrolimus (Tac), an antimetabolite [azathioprine or mycophenolate mofetil (MMF)], and a steroid in all patients. Currently, triple therapy with Tac, MMF, and steroids is the mainstream [507 out of 625 patients (81%)]. Everolimus has not been used from the early stage and has been used instead

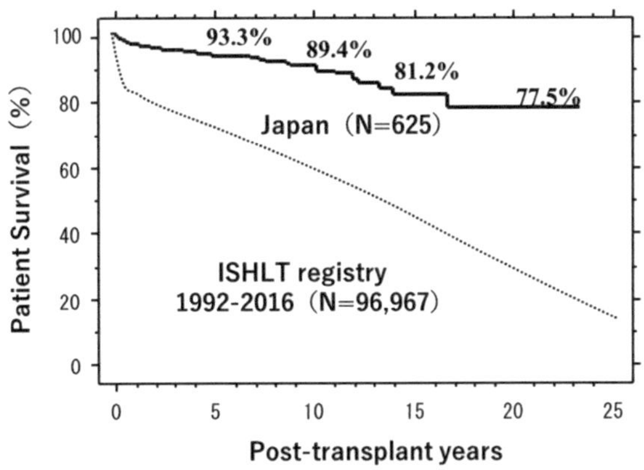

Figure 5.
Cumulative survival rate of heart transplant recipients (up to December 31, 2021). ISHLT, International Society for Heart and Lung Transplantation.

of MMF for post-transplantation coronary artery lesions, renal dysfunction, malignant tumors, and MMF-intolerant patients.

9.2.5 Recipient survival rate and social reintegration

The survival rates of 625 cases at 10, 15, and 20 years after transplantation are 93.5, 89.3, and 77.4%, which are better than those in the International Society for Heart and Lung Transplant (ISHLT) Registry (**Figure 5**). During the follow-up period of up to 23 years, 50 cases died, 13 cases of infectious diseases, 9 cases of malignant tumors (including PTLD and 1 case of brain tumor), 6 cases of multiple organ failure, 3 cases of fatal arrhythmia, and transplant coronary artery. 2 cases of sclerosis, 2 cases of transplant heart failure, 3 cases of sudden death, 1 case of renal failure, 1 case of traffic accident, 1 case of cerebral infarction, 1 case of hypoxemia, 1 case of right heart failure, 1 case of acute pancreatitis, acute respiratory failure 1 case, 1 case of heart failure, and 4 cases of unknown. As of the end of April 2022, 551 (96%) of the 575 survivors are outpatients.

Author details

Norihide Fukushima
Senri Kinran University, Japan

*Address all correspondence to: n-fukushima@cs.kinran.ac.jp

References

[1] Starzl TE, Marchioro TL, Vonkaulla KN, et al. Homotransplantation of the liver in humans. Surgery, Gynecology & Obstetrics. 1963;**117**:659-676

[2] Barnard CN. The operation a human cardiac transplant: An interim report of a successful operation performed at Groote Schuur hospital, Cape Town. South African Medical Journal. 1967;**41**:1271-1274

[3] Matsuda H, Fukushima H, Sawa Y, Nishimura M, Matsumiya G, Shirakura R. First brain dead donor heart transplantation under new legislation in Japan. The Japanese Journal of Thoracic and Cardiovascular Surgery. 1999;**47**:499-505

[4] Kitamura S, Nakatani T, Yagihara T, Sasako Y, Kobayashi J, Bando K, et al. Cardiac transplantation under new legislation for organ transplantation in Japan: Report of two cases. Japanese Circulation Journal. 2000;**64**:333-339

[5] Fukushima N. Revised organ transplant act and transplant surgeons. Japan Medical Association Journal. 2011;**54**:387-391

[6] Akutsu T et al. Permanent substitutes for valves and heart. Transactions - American Society for Artificial Internal Organs. 1958;**4**:230-235

[7] Kusserow BK. The use of a magnetic field to remotely power an implantable blood pump. Preliminary report. Transactions - American Society for Artificial Internal Organs. 1960;**4**(6):292-298

[8] Takano H, Taenaka Y, Nakatani T, et al. Circulation control of experimental and clinical profound left ventricular failures by automatic left ventricular assist system. Japanese Circulation Journal. 1984;**48**(3):302-311

[9] Fukushima N, Ono M, Saiki Y, et al. Registry report on heart transplantation in Japan (June 2016). Circulation Journal. 2017;**81**(3):298-303

[10] Fukushima N, Ono M, Nakatani T, Minami M, Konaka S, Ashikari J. Strategies for maximizing heart and lung transplantation opportunities in Japan. Transplantation Proceedings. 2009;**41**:273-276

[11] Hoefer D, Ruttmann E, Poelzl G, et al. Outcome evaluation of the bridge-to-bridge concept in patients with cardiogenic shock. The Annals of Thoracic Surgery. 2006;**82**:28-33

[12] Kitamura S, Nakatani T, Bando K, Sasako Y, Kobayashi J, Yagihara T. Modification of bicaval anastomosis technique for orthotopic heart transplantation. The Annals of Thoracic Surgery. 2001;**72**:1405-1406